T0323473

Stahl's Self-Assessment Examination in Psychiatry

Fourth edition

Stahl's Self-Assessment Examination in Psychiatry
Multiple Choice Questions for Clinicians

Fourth edition

Stephen M. Stahl
Adjunct Professor of Psychiatry,
University of California San Diego

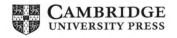

CAMBRIDGE
UNIVERSITY PRESS

University Printing House, Cambridge CB2 8BS, United Kingdom

One Liberty Plaza, 20th Floor, New York, NY 10006, USA

477 Williamstown Road, Port Melbourne, VIC 3207, Australia

314–321, 3rd Floor, Plot 3, Splendor Forum, Jasola District Centre,
New Delhi – 110025, India

103 Penang Road, #05–06/07, Visioncrest Commercial, Singapore 238467

Cambridge University Press is part of the University of Cambridge.

It furthers the University's mission by disseminating knowledge in the pursuit of
education, learning, and research at the highest international levels of excellence.

www.cambridge.org
Information on this title: www.cambridge.org/9781009241601
DOI: 10.1017/9781009241595

First published 2012
Second edition 2016
Third edition 2019
Fourth edition 2022

A catalogue record for this publication is available from the British Library.

ISBN 978-1-009-24160-1 Paperback

CONTENTS

INTRODUCTION/PREFACE

As many readers know, *Stahl's Essential Psychopharmacology* started in 1996 as a textbook (currently in its fifth edition) on **how psychotropic drugs work** and then expanded to a companion *Stahl's Prescriber's Guide* in 2005 (currently in its seventh edition) on **how to prescribe psychotropic drugs**. In 2008, a website was added (*stahlonline.org*) with both of these books available online in combination with several more, including an *Illustrated* series of several books covering specialty topics in psychopharmacology. In 2011 a case book series was added, called *Case Studies: Stahl's Essential Psychopharmacology* (now with three volumes and more to come), that shows **how to apply the concepts** presented in these previous books **to real patients in a clinical practice setting**. Now comes the fourth edition of a comprehensive set of questions and answers that we call *Stahl's Self-Assessment Examination in Psychiatry: Multiple Choice Questions for Clinicians*, designed to be integrated into the suite of our mental health/psychopharmacology books and products in the manner that I will explain here.

Why a question book?

Classically, test questions are used to measure learning, and the questions in this new book can certainly be used in this traditional manner, both by teachers and by students, and especially in combination with the companion textbook in this suite of educational products, *Stahl's Essential Psychopharmacology*. That is, teachers may wish to test student learning following their lectures on these topics by utilizing these questions and answers as part of a final examination. Also, readers not taking a formal course may wish to quiz themselves after studying specific topics in the specific chapters of the textbook. The reader will also note that documentation of the answers to each question in this book refers the reader back to the specific section of the textbook where that answer can be found and explained in great detail; outside references for the answers to the questions in the book are also provided.

Do questions just document learning?

For the modern self-directed learner, questions do much more than just document learning; they can also provide beacons for what needs to be studied and the motivation for doing that even before you read a textbook. Thus, questions are also tools for pre-study self-assessment. If you want to know whether you have already mastered a certain area of psychopharmacology, you can ask yourself these self-assessment questions BEFORE you review any specific area in the field. Many reading a textbook of psychopharmacology are not novices, but lifelong learners, and are likely to have areas of strength as well as areas of weakness. Getting correct answers will show you that a specific area is already well understood. On the other hand, getting lots of incorrect answers not only informs the self-motivated learner that a specific area needs further study, but can provide the motivation for that learner to fill in the gaps. Failure can be a powerful focuser for what to study and an energizing motivator for why to study.

"Adults don't want answers to questions they have not asked"

The truth of this old saying is that taking a test AFTER study tends to feel like being forced to answer questions that the teacher has asked. However, modern readers with the mind-set of a self-directed learner want to focus on gaps in their knowledge, so looking at these same questions PRIOR to study is a way of asking the questions of yourself and thus owning them and their answers.

What is a "knowledge sandwich?"

Ideally, self-directed learners organize their study as a "knowledge sandwich" of meaty information lying between two slices of questions. The questions in this book can be the first slice of questioning, followed by consuming the "meat" of the subject material in any textbook, including *Stahl's Essential Psychopharmacology*, or if you prefer, from a lecture, course, journal article, etc. At the end of studying, another slice of testing shows whether learning has occurred, and whether performance has improved. You can utilize, for example, the continuing medical education (CME) tests that accompany *Stahl's Essential Psychopharmacology* to test yourself after studying and document your learning (available at *neiglobal. com*). The rationale for this instructional design is also discussed in another one of our books, *Best Practices in Medical Teaching*, published in 2011. The self-assessment questions, additional "meaty" content on all the subject areas, plus posttests are also available as the "Master Psychopharmacology Program" at *neiglobal.com* for those who prefer online learning rather than a textbook.

Recertification/maintenance of certification by the American Board of Psychiatry and Neurology (ABPN)

Utilizing self-assessment questions as the first "slice" of the learning "sandwich" is not just theoretical, but is gaining prominence among expert educators these days, and indeed is now part of the requirements for maintenance of certification (MOC) in a medical specialty in the USA, including by the ABPN, which has accepted the questions in this book not only for ABPN CME requirements but also for their SA/self-assessment activity requirement, a sort of pretest.

Is your learning unforgettable?

Finally, and perhaps most importantly, tests prevent forgetting. Thus, the self-assessment questions here actually create long-term remembering, and do not just document that initial learning has occurred. It is a sorry fact that learning that occurs following one exposure/reading of material is rapidly forgotten. We have discussed this in the accompanying book in this series *Best Practices in Medical Teaching*. Perhaps 50% of what you learn after a single exposure to new, complex information is forgotten in 3–8 days, with some studies suggesting that little or nothing is remembered in 2 months! Exposing yourself to new material over time in bite-sized chunks and encountering the material again at a later time leads to more retention of information than does learning in a large bolus in a single setting, a concept sometimes called interval learning or spaced learning. Research has shown that when the re-exposure is done not as a review of the same material in the same manner, but as a test, retention is much enhanced. This results in the most efficient way of learning because the initial encoding (reading the material or hearing the lecture the first time) is consolidated for long-term retention much more effectively and completely if the re-exposure is in the form of questions. Thus, questions help you remember, and we hope that you utilize this book to maximize the efficiency of your learning to leverage the time you are able to put into your professional development.

How do you use this book?

To use this book, simply look on every right-hand page where you will see the question appear with a multiple choice format for the answer. Read the question, answer the question either in your head, on the page, or on another piece of paper. Then, turn the page and on the left side will appear not only the correct answer, but also an explanation of why the correct answer is correct, why the incorrect answers are incorrect, and references that document the correct answers, both in the companion textbook *Stahl's Essential Psychopharmacology* and elsewhere. The reader will also see at this time what peers who have already taken this test thought was the correct answer. While taking a test, the examinee is usually curious about how (s)he is doing, how many peers get a question right, and, if the wrong answer was selected, how many peers also selected that answer wrongly. Such information can provide motivation, either as reinforcement for correct answers (yes!) or to drive the reader to understand the correct answer and never to feel the sting of missing that question again (ouch!). So, it is with the greatest wishes for your successful journey throughout psychiatry and psychopharma-cology that I present this question book to you as one of the tools for your professional development, as well as for your fascination, learning, and remembering!

Stephen M. Stahl, MD, PhD

In memory of Daniel X. Freedman, mentor, colleague, and scientific father.

CME/CE INFORMATION

Released: May 2022

CME credit expires: May 2025

The chapters of this book can be completed in any order. You are advised to read each question carefully, formulate an answer, and then review the answer/explanation on the following page. If you are interested in claiming the optional CME/CE credits for a chapter, refer to that section for instructions.

Learning objectives

After completing the ten Self-Assessments, you should have identified which areas you need further study in, and be better able to:

- Apply evidence-based standards to the diagnosis of patients presenting with psychiatric symptoms to improve patient outcomes

- Prescribe treatment by linking the mechanisms of psychotropic medications to the clinical neuropathology in order to optimize response

- Apply evidence-based standards to make treatment adjustments as needed to improve patient outcomes

Optional CME/CE credits

The optional CME/CE credits are available online for a fee (waived for NEI Members). A posttest score of 70% or higher is required to receive credit. *NOTE: the questions within the assessments are not part of the posttest and do not count toward your passing score.*

For participant ease, each Self-Assessment has its own credits certificate. To receive a certificate of CME/CE credit or participation:

1. **Successfully complete a chapter posttest**: *available online at* ***neiglobal.com/CME*** *(under "Book")*

2. **Print the chapter certificate**

3. **Repeat steps 1 and 2 for each chapter**

Credit Types. The following are being offered for this activity:

- MOC SA (ABPN): Category 1 CME as Self-Assessment credits

- Nurse Practitioner (ANCC): contact hours

- Pharmacy (ACPE): application- and practice-based contact hours

- Physician (ACCME): *AMA PRA Category 1 Credits* ™

- Physician Assistant (AAPA): Category 1 CME credits

- Psychology (APA): CE credits

- Social Work (ASWB-ACE): ACE CE credits

- Non-Physician Member of the Healthcare Team: Certificate of Participation stating the program is designated for *AMA PRA Category 1 Credits* ™

MOC SA (Self Assessment) Credits Information: Any chapter posttest with a score of 70% or higher is eligible for MOC SA credits. NEI annually provides the ABPN with a report listing all successful completions.

Accreditation

In support of improving patient care, Neuroscience Education Institute (NEI) is jointly accredited by the Accreditation Council for Continuing Medical Education (ACCME), the Accreditation Council for Pharmacy Education (ACPE), and the American Nurses Credentialing Center (ANCC), to provide continuing education for the healthcare team.

NEI designates this enduring material (ten Self-Assessments) for a maximum of 16.0 *AMA PRA Category 1 Credits* ™. Physicians should claim only the credit commensurate with the extent of their participation in the activity.

The content in this activity pertains to pharmacology and is worth 16.0 continuing education hours of pharmacotherapeutics.

ABPN – Continuing Certification/Maintenance of Certification Progarm (CC/MOC): The American Board of Psychiatry and Neurology (ABPN) has reviewed *Stahl's Self-Assessment Examination in Psychiatry: Multiple Choice Questions for Clinicians, Fourth Edition* enduring material and has approved this program as part of a comprehensive lifelong learning and self-assessment program, which is mandated by the American Board of Medical

Specialties (ABMS) as a necessary component of maintenance of certification. This activity (the full book) awards *16.0 Self-Assessment Category-1 CME credits.*

Peer review

The content has been peer-reviewed by one of four MDs specializing in psychiatry (excepting "Dementia and Its Treatment," peer-reviewed by a PhD specializing in dementia) to ensure the scientific accuracy and medical relevance of information presented and its independence from bias. NEI takes responsibility for the content, quality, and scientific integrity of this CME/CE activity.

Disclosures

All individuals in a position to influence or control content were required to disclose any relevant financial relationships, which were then mitigated prior to the activity being planned, created, and presented.

Authors

Gabriela Alarcón, PhD
Medical Writer, Neuroscience Education Institute, Carlsbad, CA
No financial relationships to disclose.

Sabrina K. Bradbury-Segal, PhD
Medical Writer, Neuroscience Education Institute, Carlsbad, CA
No financial relationships to disclose.

Meghan M. Grady, BA
Vice President, Content Development, Neuroscience Education Institute, Carlsbad, CA
No financial relationships to disclose.

Elizabeth S. Lukins, BS
Medical Writer, Neuroscience Education Institute, Carlsbad, CA
No financial relationships to disclose.

Debbi A. Morrissette, PhD
Director of Content – Live Events, Neuroscience Education Institute, Carlsbad, CA
No financial relationships to disclose.

The **Planning Committee, Content Editor,** and **Peer Reviewers** have no financial relationships to disclose.

Disclosure of off-label use

This educational activity may include discussion of unlabeled and/or investigational uses of agents that are not currently labeled for such use by the US Food and Drug Administration (FDA). Please consult the product prescribing information for full disclosure of labeled uses.

Cultural linguistic competencies and implicit bias

A variety of resources addressing cultural and linguistic competencies and implicit bias can be found here: https://nei.global/CLC-IB-handout

Support

This activity is supported solely by the provider, NEI.

1 ADHD AND ITS TREATMENT

QUESTION ONE

Peter, a 35-year-old stockbroker, has been advised by his supervisor to come and see you, the company mental health consultant. His supervisor is complaining that he often comes to appointments late, is inappropriately fidgety, interrupts people during meetings, has been offensive toward coworkers, and has been known to party excessively on weeknights. Peter asserts that he is just fine; he has a lot of projects on his mind and is simply standing up for himself when speaking with others. He likes to go out in the evenings to unwind. Recognizing probable attention deficit hyperactivity disorder (ADHD), you interview both the patient and his work buddy, who is a longtime friend. How would you start your questions?

A. Compared to his parents, how often does the patient …

B. Compared to other people his age, how often does the patient …

C. Compared to his childhood, how often does the patient …

D. Compared to his children, how often does the patient …

Answer to Question One

The correct answer is B.

Choice	Peer answers
Compared to his parents, how often does the patient ...	1%
Compared to other people his age, how often does the patient ...	82%
Compared to his childhood, how often does the patient ...	17%
Compared to his children, how often does the patient ...	0%

The symptoms of ADHD can **present differently** in patients at **different ages**. While **hyperactivity** is a main symptom in children for example, this will frequently translate into **internal restlessness** in adults.

A and D – Incorrect. While ADHD has a strong genetic component, it is not advised to ask him first to compare himself to either his children or his parents. An accurate family history would be beneficial, however.

B – Correct. When trying to diagnose this adult patient with ADHD, it is preferable to **first** ask him to **compare his behavior** to that of **other adults his age**, as this will give a better idea of the severity of his symptoms at this time.

C – Incorrect. While it is important to obtain a medical history, the patient might not have the best recollection and might not be the best judge of his behaviors as a child.

Reference
Stahl SM. *Stahl's essential psychopharmacology*, fifth edition. New York, NY: Cambridge University Press; 2021. (Chapter 11)

QUESTION TWO

According to DSM-5 criteria, what is the maximum age threshold for symptom onset when making a diagnosis of ADHD?

A. 5

B. 7

C. 12

D. 15

ADHD and Its Treatment

Answer to Question Two

The correct answer is C.

Choice	Peer answers
5	4%
7	10%
12	79%
15	7%

C – Correct. In the fifth edition of the *Diagnostic and Statistical Manual of Mental Disorders*, the maximum age threshold for symptom onset for diagnosing ADHD changed from 7 to 12. Other revisions included the fact that, although symptoms must have been present prior to age 12, there does not have to have been impairment prior to age 12 when diagnosing someone who is older. The symptom count threshold also changed for adults (defined as age 17 and older), with five (instead of six) symptoms required in the inattention and/or hyperactive/impulsive categories.

A, B, and D – Incorrect.

Reference
American Psychiatric Association. *Diagnostic and statistical manual of mental disorder*, fifth edition. Arlington, VA: American Psychiatric Publishing; 2013.

QUESTION THREE

A 15-year-old with inattentive-type ADHD has a hard time staying focused on the task at hand, has trouble organizing her work, and relies heavily on her mother to follow through with her homework. Problem solving is one of the hardest tasks for her. Her difficulty with sustained attention could be related to aberrant activation in the:

A. Dorsolateral prefrontal cortex

B. Prefrontal motor cortex

C. Orbital frontal cortex

D. Supplementary motor cortex

Answer to Question Three

The correct answer is A.

Choice	Peer answers
Dorsolateral prefrontal cortex	68%
Prefrontal motor cortex	24%
Orbital frontal cortex	7%
Supplementary motor cortex	1%

A – Correct. **Sustained attention** is hypothetically modulated by the cortico-striatal-thalamic-cortical loop involving the **dorsolateral prefrontal cortex** (DLPFC). Inefficient activation of the DLPFC can lead to problems following through or finishing tasks, disorganization, and trouble sustaining mental effort; the patient exhibits all these symptoms. The dorsal **anterior cingulate cortex** is important in regulating **selective attention**, and is associated with behaviors such as losing things, being distracted, and making careless mistakes. This area is certainly also inefficient in this patient.

B – Incorrect. The **prefrontal motor cortex** hypothetically modulates behaviors such as fidgeting, leaving one's seat, running/climbing, having trouble being quiet.

C – Incorrect. The **orbital frontal cortex** regulates impulsivity, which includes symptoms such as talking excessively, blurting things out, and interrupting others.

D – Incorrect. Finally, the **supplementary motor area** is implicated in planning motor actions; thus, this brain area would be more involved in hyperactive symptoms.

References

Arnsten AF. Fundamentals of attention-deficit/hyperactivity disorder: circuits and pathways. *J Clin Psychiatry* 2006;67(Suppl 8):7–12.

Stahl SM. *Stahl's essential psychopharmacology*, fifth edition. New York, NY: Cambridge University Press; 2021. (Chapter 11)

Stahl SM, Mignon L. *Stahl's illustrated attention deficit hyperactivity disorder*. New York, NY: Cambridge University Press; 2009. (Chapter 1)

QUESTION FOUR

Which of the following is true regarding cortical brain development in children with ADHD compared to healthy controls?

A. The pattern (i.e., order) of cortical maturation is different

B. The timing of cortical maturation is different

C. The pattern and timing of cortical maturation are different

D. Neither the pattern nor the timing of cortical maturation is different

ADHD and Its Treatment

Answer to Question Four

The correct answer is B.

Choice	Peer answers
The pattern (i.e., order) of cortical maturation is different	8%
The timing of cortical maturation is different	34%
The pattern and timing of cortical maturation are different	52%
Neither the pattern nor the timing of cortical maturation is different	6%

ADHD is a neurodevelopmental disorder characterized by inattentive, hyperactive, and/or impulsive symptoms. Neuroimaging has been used to evaluate cortical maturation in children with ADHD compared to typically developing controls, specifically by comparing the age of attaining peak cortical thickness in children with and without ADHD.

A – Incorrect. Research shows that the pattern of cortical maturation is similar for children with and without ADHD. Specifically, the primary sensory and motor areas attain peak cortical thickness earlier in development than do high-order association areas such as the dorsolateral prefrontal cortex.

B – Correct. There are differences in the timing of cortical maturation between children with and without ADHD that are apparent as early as age 7. That is, cortical maturation in children with ADHD seems to lag behind that of healthy children. In fact, the median age by which 50% of the cortical points achieve peak thickness is delayed by 3 years in children with ADHD. Delay is most prominent in the superior and dorsolateral prefrontal regions, which are particularly important for control of attention and planning. Delay is also seen in subcortical structures. A large cross-sectional mega-analysis demonstrated that the delay in brain maturation is not attributable to medication use.

Interestingly, there is one brain region in which children with ADHD achieve peak cortical thickness earlier than typically developing controls: the primary motor cortex.

C and D – Incorrect.

ADHD and Its Treatment

References

Hoogman M, Bralten J, Hibar DP et al. Subcortical brain volume differences in participants with attention deficit hyperactivity disorder in children and adults: a cross-sectional mega-analysis. *Lancet Psychiatry* 2017;4(4):310–19.

Shaw P, Eckstrand K, Sharp W et al. Attention-deficit/hyperactivity disorder is characterized by a delay in cortical maturation. *Proc Natl Acad Sci U S A* 2007;104(49):19649–54.

ADHD and Its Treatment

QUESTION FIVE

Irina is a 35-year-old patient with untreated ADHD who reports abusing alcohol to manage severe anxiety. Irina's symptoms may represent a case where the firing of _____ and _____ neurons innervating her prefrontal cortex is dysregulated and causing excessive arousal.

A. Norepinephrine; glutamate

B. Norepinephrine; dopamine

C. Dopamine; glutamate

D. Dopamine; serotonin

ADHD and Its Treatment

Answer to Question Five

The correct answer is B.

Choice	Peer answers
Norepinephrine; glutamate	23%
Norepinephrine; dopamine	57%
Dopamine; glutamate	16%
Dopamine; serotonin	5%

A – Incorrect.

B – Correct. When norepinephrine (NE) and dopamine (DA) neurotransmission in the prefrontal cortex are optimally tuned, modest stimulation of postsynaptic alpha 2A receptors and dopamine 1 receptors allows for efficient cognitive functioning. If NE or DA neurotransmission is excessive, as in situations of stress or comorbid conditions such as anxiety or substance abuse, this can lead to overstimulation of postsynaptic receptors and consequently to cognitive dysfunction as well as other symptoms.

C – Incorrect.

D – Incorrect.

Reference
Stahl SM. *Stahl's essential psychopharmacology*, fifth edition. New York, NY: Cambridge University Press; 2021. (Chapter 11)

QUESTION SIX

Martin is a 19-year-old patient with a history of ADHD since childhood and is treated with an immediate-release amphetamine (D, L) tablet once a day upon waking. However, Martin has now started college and his class schedule is spread out throughout the day. He complains that he is unable to concentrate and takes scattered notes during his early evening courses. What dose adjustment would you recommend?

A. Decrease the dose of his immediate-release amphetamine

B. Increase the dose of his immediate-release amphetamine

C. Switch to an extended-release formulation of amphetamine

D. Do not change anything

ADHD and Its Treatment

Answer to Question Six

The correct answer is C.

Choice	Peer answers
Decrease the dose of his immediate-release amphetamine	0%
Increase the dose of his immediate-release amphetamine	1%
Switch to an extended-release formulation of amphetamine	99%
Do not change anything	0%

The goal is to enhance phasic DA neurotransmission with low to moderate, continuous drug delivery, trying to increase mostly tonic DA firing and only judiciously increase phasic DA firing. To achieve prudent and therapeutic improvement of tonic and phasic DA neurotransmission, without disastrous increases in phasic DA neurotransmission leading to abuse and addiction, sustained delivery is what is wanted.

A – Incorrect. Immediate-release preparations have a duration of 4–6 hours. Decreasing the dose of immediate-release amphetamine (D, L) will have no therapeutic effect on helping the patient manage his symptoms later in the day.

B – Incorrect. Immediate-release preparations have a duration of 4–6 hours. Pharmacological actions of high-dose amphetamine are not linked to therapeutic action in ADHD, but to reinforcement, reward, and euphoria in amphetamine abuse. Increasing the dose of immediate-release formulations elicits pulsatile drug administration that causes immediate release of DA and could potentially lead to the highly reinforcing pleasurable effects of drug abuse, especially at high enough doses and rapid enough administration. For this reason, using immediate-release stimulants, especially in young adults, is increasingly being avoided.

C – Correct. Extended-release preparations have a duration ranging from 8 to 16 hours, depending on the formulation. Controlled-release (or extended-release) preparations for stimulants result in slowly rising, constant, steady-state levels of the drug. Under those circumstances, the firing pattern of DA will theoretically be mostly tonic, regular, and not at the mercy of fluctuating levels of DA. Some pulsatile firing is fine, especially when involved in reinforcing learning and salience.

D – Incorrect. Not changing anything will have no therapeutic effect on helping the patient manage his symptoms later in the day.

References

Cortese S, Adamo N, Del Giovane C et al. Comparative efficacy and tolerability of medications for attention-deficit hyperactivity disorder in children, adolescents, and adults: a systematic review and network meta-analysis. *Lancet Psychiatry* 2018;5(9):727–38.

Stahl SM. *Stahl's essential psychopharmacology*, fifth edition. New York, NY: Cambridge University Press; 2021. (Chapter 11)

ADHD and Its Treatment

QUESTION SEVEN

Alexandra, a 27-year-old bartender, was diagnosed with ADHD at age 10. She has been on and off medication since then, first on immediate-release methylphenidate, then on the methylphenidate patch. She experimented with illicit drugs during her late adolescence and is still a heavy drinker. After a few years of self-medication with alcohol and cigarettes, she is seeking medical attention again. You decide to put her on 80 mg/day of atomoxetine, one of the nonstimulant medications effective in ADHD. Why does atomoxetine lack abuse potential?

A. It decreases norepinephrine levels in the nucleus accumbens, but not in the prefrontal cortex

B. It increases dopamine levels in the prefrontal cortex but not in the nucleus accumbens

C. It modulates serotonin levels in the raphe nucleus

D. It increases dopamine in the striatum and anterior cingulate cortex

ADHD and Its Treatment

Answer to Question Seven

The correct answer is B.

Choice	Peer answers
It decreases norepinephrine levels in the nucleus accumbens, but not in the prefrontal cortex	17%
It increases dopamine levels in the prefrontal cortex but not in the nucleus accumbens	69%
It modulates serotonin levels in the raphe nucleus	9%
It increases dopamine in the striatum and anterior cingulate cortex	5%

Atomoxetine is a selective norepinephrine reuptake inhibitor (**NET inhibitor**).

A – Incorrect. In the nucleus accumbens there are only a few NE neurons and NE transporters. **Inhibiting NET in the nucleus accumbens** will not lead to an increase in NE or DA.

B – Correct. The prefrontal cortex lacks high concentrations of dopamine transporter (DAT), so in this brain region, DA gets inactivated by NET. Therefore, **inhibiting NET in the prefrontal cortex** increases both DA and NE. As only a few NET exist in the nucleus accumbens, atomoxetine does not induce an increase in DA and NE in the nucleus accumbens, the reward center of the brain, thus atomoxetine does not have abuse potential.

C – Incorrect. Atomoxetine does not modulate serotonin levels.

D – Incorrect. The striatum and the anterior cingulate cortex are not brain areas involved in reward.

Reference

Stahl SM. *Stahl's essential psychopharmacology*, fifth edition. New York, NY: Cambridge University Press; 2021. (Chapter 11)

QUESTION EIGHT

A 14-year-old patient with ADHD has a rare mutation in the gene for the dopamine transporter (DAT). In deciding which treatment to initiate for this patient's ADHD, you know it will be important to avoid treatments that depend on normally functioning DAT. Which of the following drugs are transported into neurons via the DAT?

A. Methylphenidate

B. Atomoxetine

C. Amphetamine

Answer to Question Eight

The correct answer is C.

Choice	Peer answers
Methylphenidate	15%
Atomoxetine	23%
Amphetamine	62%

A – Incorrect. Methylphenidate binds to the DAT and to the norepinephrine transporter (NET), in both cases acting as an allosteric modulator. That is, it binds to each transporter at a different site than the neurotransmitter itself binds. When it does so, it stops the action of the transporters, preventing reuptake and thus allowing DA and NE to accumulate in the synapse. Methylphenidate itself is not taken up into the presynaptic neuron.

B – Incorrect. Atomoxetine is an inhibitor of the NET, and like methylphenidate it binds at a site distinct from where monoamines bind. It does not have actions at the DAT.

C – Correct. Like methylphenidate, amphetamine blocks the transporters for both DA and NE. However, unlike methylphenidate, which acts as an allosteric modulator, amphetamine is a pseudo-substrate and a competitive inhibitor at these receptors. That is, it binds to the same site as the substrate – either DA or NE – thus competing with the neurotransmitters and preventing them from being taken up into the terminal. In addition, because amphetamine is a pseudosubstrate, it is actually transported into the presynaptic nerve terminal. This is important, because amphetamine is *also* a pseudosubstrate and competitive inhibitor at the vesicular monoamine transporter (VMAT). VMAT is a proton pump that exchanges DA for protons, packaging the DA into synaptic vesicles where it is stored for subsequent reuse. When amphetamine binds to VMAT, it not only blocks the further transport of DA into synaptic vesicles but is actually packaged into vesicles itself, where it has the ability to displace stored DA – or NE – back into the cytoplasm. This occurs only at high doses of amphetamine, as in cases of amphetamine abuse.

Reference
Stahl SM. *Stahl's essential psychopharmacology*, fifth edition. New York, NY: Cambridge University Press; 2021. (Chapter 11)

QUESTION NINE

A patient with ADHD has not yet had successful treatment: he has experienced either loss of efficacy toward the end of the day or efficacy but insomnia at night. He is frustrated and wants to know what other treatment options exist. The most recently available new treatments for ADHD represent:

A. Novel neurotransmitter targets

B. New formulations of existing active ingredients

Answer to Question Nine

The correct answer is B.

Choice	Peer answers
Novel neurotransmitter targets	21%
New formulations of existing active ingredients	79%

A – Incorrect. Investigational and recently available medications for ADHD largely still target the DA and/or NE system.

B – Correct. The majority of approved treatments for ADHD, and specifically new agents approved recently, are formulation variations of either amphetamine or methylphenidate. Their differences lie not in the active ingredient but rather in how that active ingredient is delivered (i.e., release mechanism). Modified-release formulations are designed to release the drug in a controlled and predictable manner that allows for a particular efficacy and safety profile. Modifying the release of the drug can improve tolerability by eliminating peaks and troughs in plasma concentration and can improve efficacy by increasing duration of action as well as by eliminating peaks and troughs.

References

Grady MM, Stahl SM. A horse of a different color: how formulation influences medication effects. *CNS Spectr* 2012;17:63–9.

Neuroscience Education Institute. NEI Prescribe [Mobile application software]. 2020. Available at: http://nei.global/neiprescribeitunes.

ADHD and Its Treatment

QUESTION TEN

Rita is a 28-year-old patient with untreated ADHD. You are currently deciding between guanfacine and clonidine as potential treatments for this patient. The selective alpha 2A agonist guanfacine appears to be:

A. Less tolerated than the alpha 2 agonist clonidine

B. Better tolerated than the alpha 2 agonist clonidine

C. Less efficacious than the alpha 2 agonist clonidine

D. More efficacious than the alpha 2 agonist clonidine

ADHD and Its Treatment

Answer to Question Ten

The correct answer is B.

Choice	Peer answers
Less tolerated than the alpha 2 agonist clonidine	4%
Better tolerated than the alpha 2 agonist clonidine	75%
Less efficacious than the alpha 2 agonist clonidine	6%
More efficacious than the alpha 2 agonist clonidine	15%

There are two direct-acting agonists for alpha 2 receptors used to treat ADHD, guanfacine and clonidine. Guanfacine is relatively more selective for alpha 2A receptors than for other subtypes, whereas clonidine binds to alpha 2A, alpha 2B, and alpha 2C receptors. Clonidine also has actions on imidazoline receptors, which is thought to be responsible for some of clonidine's sedating and hypotensive actions.

A – Incorrect. Although the actions of clonidine at alpha 2A receptors exhibit therapeutic potential for ADHD, its actions at other receptors may increase side effects. By contrast, guanfacine is 15–60 times more selective for alpha 2A receptors than for alpha 2B and alpha 2C receptors. Additionally, guanfacine is ten times weaker than clonidine at inducing sedation and lowering blood pressure. Thus, guanfacine is better tolerated than clonidine.

B – Correct. Guanfacine is better tolerated than clonidine.

C – Incorrect. Guanfacine is 25 times more potent in enhancing prefrontal cortical function. Thus, it can be said that guanfacine exhibits therapeutic efficacy with a reduced side effect profile compared to clonidine.

D – Incorrect. There are no head-to-head comparisons to establish that guanfacine has superior efficacy to clonidine in ADHD.

References

Stahl SM. *Stahl's essential psychopharmacology, the prescriber's guide*, seventh edition. New York, NY: Cambridge University Press; 2020.

Stahl SM. *Stahl's essential psychopharmacology*, fifth edition. New York, NY: Cambridge University Press; 2021. (Chapter 11)

QUESTION ELEVEN

Aggregate data suggest that, compared to stimulants, nonstimulants have:

A. Smaller effect sizes

B. Approximately the same effect sizes

C. Larger effect sizes

ADHD and Its Treatment

Answer to Question Eleven

The correct answer is A.

Choice	Peer answers
Smaller effect sizes	82%
Approximately the same effect sizes	16%
Larger effect sizes	2%

A – Correct. Multiple meta-analyses assessing the effects of stimulant medications have shown that, as a class, nonstimulants have smaller effect sizes than stimulants. Due to differences in study design, these meta-analyses do not address potential differences in efficacy among specific medications.

B and C – Incorrect.

References
Faraone SV, Glatt SJ. A comparison of the efficacy of medications for adult attention-deficit/hyperactivity disorder using meta-analysis of effect sizes. *J Clin Psychiatry* 2010;71(6):754–63.

Faraone SV, Biederman J, Spencer TJ, Aleardi M. Comparing the efficacy of medications for ADHD using meta-analysis. *MedGenMed* 2006;8(4):4.

Hanwella R, Senanayake M, de Silva V. Comparative efficacy and acceptability of methylphenidate and atomoxetine in treatment of attention deficit hyperactivity disorder in children and adolescents: a meta-analysis. *BMC Psychiatry* 2011;11:176.

ADHD and Its Treatment

QUESTION TWELVE

Isaac is an 8-year-old patient with ADHD. Among male children with ADHD, which of the following is the most commonly seen comorbidity?

A. Anxiety

B. Oppositional defiant disorder

C. Depression

STAHL'S SELF-ASSESSMENT EXAMINATION IN PSYCHIATRY

Answer to Question Twelve

The correct answer is B.

Choice	Peer answers
Anxiety	15%
Oppositional defiant disorder	81%
Depression	4%

A and C – Incorrect. While anxiety and depression are common comorbidities in patients with ADHD, they are more often found in girls compared to boys.

B – Correct. Argumentative, disobedient, and aggressive behaviors are often seen in patients suffering from ADHD and oppositional symptoms. The presence of comorbid disruptive behavior disorders such as oppositional defiant disorder, or conduct disorder, within children with ADHD has been well established. About five in ten children with ADHD have a behavior or conduct problem and this is seen at a higher rate in boys than in girls in studies.

References

Elwin M, Elvin T, Larsson JO. Symptoms and level of functioning related to comorbidity in children and adolescents with ADHD: a cross-sectional registry study. *Child Adolesc Psychiatry Ment Health* 2020;14:30.

Jensen PS, Hinshaw SP, Kraemer HC et al. ADHD comorbidity findings from the MTA study: comparing comorbid subgroups. *J Am Acad Child Adolesc Psychiatry* 2001;40(2):147–58.

Reale L, Bartoli B, Cartabia M et al. Comorbidity prevalence and treatment outcome in children and adolescents with ADHD. *Eur Child Adolesc Psychiatry* 2017;26(12):1443–57.

ADHD and Its Treatment

QUESTION THIRTEEN

A 44-year-old man was diagnosed with ADHD, inattentive sub-type, in college but has not taken medication for the last several years. He is seeking treatment now because of declining work performance following a promotion 7 months ago. Specifically, he complains of difficulty finishing papers and staying focused during meetings, and fears that his boss is losing confidence in him. Assessment confirms a diagnosis of ADHD, inattentive subtype. After 2 months of treatment on a therapeutic dose of a long-acting stimulant, he states that his focus, sustained attention, and distractibility are much better, but that he still can't get organized and that it takes him longer to complete tasks than it should. At this point, would it be appropriate to raise the dose of the stimulant to try to address his residual symptoms?

A. Yes

B. No

ADHD and Its Treatment

Answer to Question Thirteen

The correct answer is B.

Choice	Peer answers
Yes	56%
No	44%

A – Incorrect. Dose response studies of stimulant medications suggest that the optimal dose varies across individuals and depends somewhat on the domain of function. Specifically, higher doses may lead to greater improvement of some domains (e.g., vigilance, attention) but not executive function (e.g., planning, cognitive flexibility, inhibitory control).

B – Correct. If medication dose is high enough to substantially diminish symptoms of inattention and distractibility, then executive function needs to be addressed independently and will not likely respond to higher medication dosing.

References

Pietrzak RH, Mollica CM, Maruff P, Snyder PJ. Cognitive effects of immediate-release methylphenidate in children with attention-deficit/hyperactivity disorder. *Neurosci Biobehav Rev* 2006;30:1225–45.

Swanson J, Baler RD, Volkow ND. Understanding the effects of stimulant medications on cognition individuals with attention–deficit hyperactivity disorder: a decade of progress. *Neuropsychopharmacology* 2011;36:207–26.

ADHD and Its Treatment

QUESTION FOURTEEN

The cumulative data on the effects of physical exercise as an adjunctive treatment for children with ADHD have demonstrated the potential beneficial effects of:

A. Acute aerobic exercise

B. Chronic aerobic exercise

C. A and B

D. Neither A nor B

Answer to Question Fourteen

The correct answer is C.

Choice	Peer answers
Acute aerobic exercise	11%
Chronic aerobic exercise	13%
A and B	74%
Neither A nor B	3%

A and B – Partially correct.

C – Correct. Comparisons have been made between aerobic/nonaerobic, and acute vs. chronic exercise on cognitive and behavioral symptoms in children with ADHD. Numerous published studies on exercise and cognition in children with ADHD have shown that aerobic exercise appears to be the most effective for improvements in executive function. Both acute and chronic exercise have beneficial effects on behavioral and cognitive measures in children with ADHD, when assessed immediately after exercise. Cognitive measures include improved response inhibition, cognitive control, attention allocation, cognitive flexibility, processing speed, and vigilance.

Physical exercise is beneficial as adjunctive treatment, but there is not enough evidence to suggest that it is a stand-alone treatment. Exercise may be particularly effective for youth, potentially preventing or altering the course of ADHD. The literature is promising; however, the most challenging complications for these types of studies are random assignment, blinded raters, and adequate control groups.

D – Incorrect.

References

Den Heijer AE, **Groen Y**, **Tucha L** et al. Sweat it out? The effects of physical exercise on cognition and behavior in children and adults with ADHD: a systematic literature review. *J Neural Transm (Vienna)* 2017;124(Suppl 1):3–26.

Hoza B, **Martin CP**, **Pirog A** et al. Using physical activity to manage ADHD symptoms: the state of the evidence. *Curr Psychiatry Rep* 2016;18(12):113.

QUESTION FIFTEEN

A patient with a history of alcohol use disorder has been sober for 6 weeks. He begins medication treatment for adult ADHD and experiences improvement, but 4 months later relapses with his alcohol use disorder, engaging in three binge drinking episodes over a 2-week period. Does this patient need to discontinue medication treatment for ADHD?

A. Yes, he should be switched to a non-medication treatment

B. Only if he is currently on a long-acting stimulant; nonstimulant medication is acceptable in this scenario

C. No, both long-acting stimulants and nonstimulant medications are acceptable in this scenario

ADHD and Its Treatment

Answer to Question Fifteen

The correct answer is C.

Choice	Peer answers
Yes, he should be switched to a non-medication treatment	11%
Only if he is currently on a long-acting stimulant; nonstimulant medication is acceptable in this scenario	32%
No, both long-acting stimulants and nonstimulant medications are acceptable in this scenario	58%

A – Incorrect. Because ongoing substance abuse can hinder the treatment progress of other disorders, in many cases it may be necessary to address this problem first. However, these are general guidelines in the ordering of treatment, and one should be careful that this prioritization of symptoms/conditions does not lead to the neglect of ADHD treatment in adults. In fact, there is an evidence base for prescribing ADHD medication for patients in early sobriety from an alcohol use disorder. Specifically, atomoxetine, which is approved for adult ADHD, has been shown to be effective for ADHD and to decrease both alcohol cravings and heavy drinking days. Atomoxetine is not contraindicated in patients with acute alcohol use disorder or in patients with liver impairment, so the patient's alcohol use would not require medication discontinuation. It is an appropriate treatment choice; however, it is not the only appropriate treatment choice.

B – Incorrect. Long-acting stimulant medications are not contraindicated in patients with acute alcohol use disorder, although they do carry a black box warning indicating caution in patients with a history of substance dependence. In general, nonstimulant options may be preferable to stimulants in patients with substance use disorders, but long-acting stimulants should remain as a second-tier option.

C – Correct. Nonstimulant and long-acting stimulant medications are both options for ADHD co-occurring with substance use disorders; however, nonstimulants may be preferred as the first-line approach. If a stimulant is prescribed to a patient in early sobriety from substance use and/or continued low-level substance use, then he/she should be monitored closely for misuse of the prescribed medication.

References

McGough JJ. Treatment controversies in adult ADHD. *Am J Psychiatry* 2016;173:960–6.

Wilens TE, Morrison NR. The intersection of attention-deficit/hyperactivity disorder and substance abuse. *Curr Opin Psychiatry* 2011;24:280–5.

Wilens TE, Morrison NR, Prince J. An update on the pharmacotherapy of attention-deficit/hyperactivity disorder in adults. *Expert Rev Neurother* 2011;11(10):1443–65.

ADHD and Its Treatment

QUESTION SIXTEEN

A 7-year-old boy has just been diagnosed with ADHD, combined type, and his care provider feels that the best therapeutic choice is a stimulant. Family history is significant for depression and diabetes. The patient's medical history is significant for asthma; physical exam reveals no abnormalities. According to current recommendations, what should be the care provider's next step?

A. Prescribe a stimulant, as no additional tests are indicated for this patient

B. Obtain an electrocardiogram (ECG), as this patient's family history and exam results warrant it

C. Obtain an ECG, as this is mandatory prior to prescribing a stimulant to any child

D. Prescribe a nonstimulant, as a stimulant would not be appropriate for this patient

Answer to Question Sixteen

The correct answer is A.

Choice	Peer answers
Prescribe a stimulant, as no additional tests are indicated for this patient	71%
Obtain an electrocardiogram (ECG), as this patient's family history and exam results warrant it	8%
Obtain an ECG, as this is mandatory prior to prescribing a stimulant to any child	17%
Prescribe a nonstimulant, as a stimulant would not be appropriate for this patient	4%

A – Correct. Current recommendations from the American Heart Association (AHA) are that it is reasonable but not mandatory to obtain an ECG prior to prescribing a stimulant to a child. The American Academy of Pediatrics (AAP) does not recommend an ECG prior to starting a stimulant for most children.

B – Incorrect. According to recommendations, it is at the physician's discretion whether to obtain an ECG; however, in this case there is no evidence of cardiovascular disease in either the family history or patient exam.

C – Incorrect. According to AHA and AAP recommendations, treatment with a stimulant should not be withheld because an ECG is not obtained.

D – Incorrect. There is no reason why a stimulant would not be a reasonable choice for this patient.

Reference

American Academy of Pediatrics/American Heart Association.
American Academy of Pediatrics/American Heart Association clarification of statement on cardiovascular evaluation and monitoring of children and adolescents with heart disease receiving medications for ADHD. *J Dev Behav Pediatr* 2008;29(4):335.

CHAPTER PEER COMPARISON

For the ADHD section, the correct answer was selected 70% of the time.

2 ANXIETY/STRESS DISORDERS AND THEIR TREATMENT

QUESTION ONE

A 35-year-old female presents to your office and begins to divulge her frequent worries: ever since she was young, she was worried someone close to her would die in a freak accident. As she grew older, this worry was exacerbated by the fear that she would pass away without telling her friends and family how important they are to her. Additionally, once she had children, she became so worried for their safety that she rarely lets them leave the house. Furthermore, she has constant worries about how things will work out for her in the future, and recently experienced a panic attack. Based only on what you know here, how might you currently diagnose this patient?

A. Posttraumatic stress disorder (PTSD)

B. Panic disorder

C. Social anxiety disorder

D. Generalized anxiety disorder

Answer to Question One

The correct answer is D.

Choice	Peer answers
Posttraumatic stress disorder (PTSD)	1%
Panic disorder	4%
Social anxiety disorder	1%
Generalized anxiety disorder	94%

A – Incorrect. PTSD generally originates after a traumatic event; it does not appear that this patient has ever actually experienced a traumatic death experience. She just appears to have excessive worry.

B – Incorrect. Panic disorder is characterized by the presence of spontaneous panic attacks, which this patient does not report having.

C – Incorrect. Worry in social anxiety disorder is most often tied to fear of scrutiny by others, or embarrassing oneself, in certain social situations, whereas this patient's worry is related to a fear of dying.

D – Correct. This patient is displaying core symptoms of generalized anxiety disorder via generalized anxiety and worry. Although she did have a panic attack, a single panic attack is insufficient for a diagnosis of either panic disorder or social anxiety disorder.

References

American Psychiatric Association. *Diagnostic and statistical manual of mental disorder*, fifth edition. Arlington, VA: American Psychiatric Publishing; 2013.

Stahl SM. *Stahl's essential psychopharmacology*, fifth edition. New York, NY: Cambridge University Press; 2021. (Chapter 8)

Stahl SM, Grady MM. *Stahl's illustrated anxiety, stress, and PTSD*. New York, NY: Cambridge University Press; 2010. (Chapter 2)

QUESTION TWO

What neurocircuitry is involved in the major core symptom of worry, which occurs across the spectrum of anxiety disorders?

A. Reciprocal connections between the amygdala and anterior cingulate cortex (ACC)

B. Reciprocal connections between the amygdala and the periaqueductal gray area (PAG)

C. Cortico-striato-thalamo-cortical (CSTC) loop

D. Reciprocal connections between the amygdala and orbitofrontal cortex (OFC)

Answer to Question Two

The correct answer is C.

Choice	Peer answers
Reciprocal connections between the amygdala and anterior cingulate cortex (ACC)	35%
Reciprocal connections between the amygdala and the periaqueductal gray area (PAG)	4%
Cortico-striato-thalamo-cortical (CSTC) loop	41%
Reciprocal connections between the amygdala and orbitofrontal cortex (OFC)	19%

A – Incorrect. Feelings of fear, another core symptom of anxiety disorders, are regulated by reciprocal connections between the amygdala and the ACC. Reciprocal connections between the amygdala and the OFC are also involved. Overactivation of these circuits could produce feelings of fear.

B – Incorrect. Feelings of fear may be expressed through behaviors such as avoidance, which is partly regulated by reciprocal connections between the amygdala and the PAG. Avoidance is characterized by a motor response and may be analogous to freezing under threat. Other motor responses are to fight or run away (flight) in order to survive threats from the environment.

C – Correct. Worry is regulated by a CSTC loop.

D – Incorrect. Feelings of fear are regulated by the reciprocal connections between the amygdala and the OFC. Reciprocal connections between the amygdala and the ACC are also involved. Overactivation of these circuits could produce feelings of fear.

References

Stahl SM. *Stahl's essential psychopharmacology*, fifth edition. New York, NY: Cambridge University Press; 2021. (Chapter 8)

Stahl SM, Grady MM. *Stahl's illustrated anxiety, stress, and PTSD*. New York, NY: Cambridge University Press; 2010. (Chapter 2)

QUESTION THREE

A 46-year-old female patient has been experiencing several anxiety-based symptoms for many years and was previously diagnosed with generalized anxiety disorder. She describes difficulty concentrating in addition to difficulty falling asleep. Her family has recently told her that she seems to be displaying heightened anger responses toward them over minor details. Oftentimes she will cry for extended periods of time and become irritable and distant. Based on the above patient's revelations, if she were to continue to experience these stressful reactions to stimuli (i.e., excessive crying, fatigue, problems concentrating, tension, irritability), what could potentially occur?

A. Increased hippocampal volume

B. Reduced brain-derived neurotrophic factor (BDNF) production

C. Reduced reactivity to stress

D. Decreased hippocampal volume

E. B and D

F. A and C

Answer to Question Three

The correct answer is E.

Choice	Peer answers
Increased hippocampal volume	2%
Reduced brain-derived neurotrophic factor (BDNF) production	5%
Reduced reactivity to stress	1%
Decreased hippocampal volume	4%
B and D	83%
A and C	5%

A and C – Incorrect. Hippocampal volume in chronic stress is actually theorized to decrease, not increase. Reduced reactivity to stress may occur in patients who experience mild stressors while growing up, which may result in an improved adaptability when dealing with adult stressors. However, severe or persistent stress, such as this adult is experiencing, does not lead to reduced reactivity to stress.

B and D – Correct. Reduced BDNF production can occur in patients who experience chronic stress, leading to a decreased ability to create and maintain neurons and neuronal connections. Decreased hippocampal volume, perhaps related to decreased expression of BDNF, has been reported in some chronic stress conditions, such as major depression, and certain anxiety disorders. A major treatment strategy for stress-related disorders is the use of selective serotonin reuptake inhibitors (SSRIs), which can increase BDNF levels because serotonin initiates signal transduction cascades that lead to BDNF release.

E – Correct; as both B and D are correct answers.

F – Incorrect; as both A and C are incorrect answers.

References

Bremner JD. Stress and brain atrophy. *CNS Neurol Disord Drug Targets* 2006;5(5):503–12.

Stahl SM, Grady MM. *Stahl's illustrated anxiety, stress, and PTSD*. New York, NY: Cambridge University Press; 2010. (Chapter 1)

QUESTION FOUR

A 51-year-old male veteran with chronic PTSD has agreed to begin pharmacotherapy for his debilitating symptoms of arousal and anxiety associated with his experiences in Iraq 2 years ago. Which of the following would be appropriate as first-line treatment?

A. Paroxetine

B. Paroxetine or lorazepam

C. Paroxetine, lorazepam, or D-cycloserine

D. Paroxetine, lorazepam, D-cycloserine, or quetiapine

Anxiety/Stress Disorders and Their Treatment

Answer to Question Four

The correct answer is A.

Choice	Peer answers
Paroxetine	91%
Paroxetine or lorazepam	4%
Paroxetine, lorazepam, or D-cycloserine	2%
Paroxetine, lorazepam, D-cycloserine, or quetiapine	2%

A – Correct. Paroxetine, a selective serotonin reuptake inhibitor (SSRI), is approved for use in PTSD. The SSRI sertraline is also approved for PTSD.

B – Incorrect. Lorazepam is a benzodiazepine. Benzodiazepines do not have evidence of efficacy in PTSD and are not generally recommended for first-line use in PTSD.

C – Incorrect. D-cycloserine, an N-methyl-D-aspartate (NMDA) agonist, has been theorized to be useful in facilitating fear extinction, and may be useful in conjunction with exposure therapy. However, it is not a first-line choice.

D – Incorrect. Quetiapine, an atypical antipsychotic, is not approved as first-line treatment for PTSD but may be useful in selected cases as a third-line treatment, specifically for sleep and possible reduction of nightmares.

References

Sauvé W, Stahl SM. Psychopharmacological treatment of PTSD. In: *Treating PTSD in military personnel: a clinical handbook*. New York, NY: Guilford Press; 2011.

Stahl SM. *Case studies: Stahl's essential psychopharmacology*. New York, NY: Cambridge University Press; 2011.

Stahl SM, Grady MM. *Stahl's illustrated anxiety, stress, and PTSD*. New York, NY: Cambridge University Press; 2010. (Chapters 4–8)

Walter A. Pharmacotherapy for post-traumatic stress disorders in combat veterans? Focus on antidepressants and atypical antipsychotic agents. *P T* 2012;37(1):32–8.

QUESTION FIVE

A 38-year-old male combat veteran with chronic PTSD has agreed to begin pharmacotherapy for his debilitating symptoms of arousal and anxiety associated with his experiences in Iraq several years ago. He is the sole survivor of his battalion in a convoy attack. He was given the maximum doses of two different selective serotonin reuptake inhibitors (SSRIs), approved by the US Food and Drug Administration (FDA) for PTSD treatment, but neither alleviated his symptoms. He has wanted to try exposure therapy, but reliving the event is too much for him, and so he has avoided this therapy. He may be an excellent candidate for the use of 3,4-methylenedioxymethamphetamine (MDMA)-assisted psychotherapy. MDMA is a psychoactive substance that promotes release of serotonin, norepinephrine, and dopamine by reversing membrane-bound transporter proteins and inhibiting reuptake in the mesolimbocortical circuitry, and by stimulation of neurohormonal signaling of oxytocin, cortisol, prolactin, and vasopressin. The underlying mechanism for this type of treatment is based on:

A. Enhanced dopamine may underlie the destabilization of memory reactivation during reconsolidation processing

B. Enhanced gamma-aminobutyric acid (GABA) may make it easy to forget traumatic memories

C. Enhanced serotonin may allow for positive affective states and prosocial effects that present a safe environment for reconsolidation to occur

D. A and C

E. B and C

Anxiety/Stress Disorders and Their Treatment

Answer to Question Five

The correct answer is D.

Choice	Peer answers
Enhanced dopamine may underlie the destabilization of memory reactivation during reconsolidation processing	2%
Enhanced gamma-aminobutyric acid (GABA) may make it easy to forget traumatic memories	1%
Enhanced serotonin may allow for positive affective states and prosocial effects that present a safe environment for reconsolidation to occur.	11%
A and C	72%
B and C	14%

A – Partially correct.

B – Incorrect. MDMA is a psychoactive substance that promotes release of serotonin, norepinephrine, and dopamine by reversing membrane-bound transporter proteins and inhibiting reuptake in the mesolimbocortical circuitry, and by stimulation of neurohormonal signaling of oxytocin, cortisol, prolactin, and vasopressin. It does not act on the GABAergic system.

C – Partially correct.

D – Correct. Dopamine signaling via ventral tegmental area (VTA) projections to the amygdala is associated with destabilization of a memory but is not involved in modification or restabilization of the trace. Once a memory becomes destabilized and labile during a therapy session, MDMA may influence activity in neurocircuitry necessary for learning and memory. Through enhanced serotonin release, MDMA can induce positive affective states and prosocial effects that signal a safe and supportive setting. Prior reconsolidation research during affective psychotherapy suggests feelings of safety are necessary for traumatic memories to be amended with less fear.

E – Incorrect.

Reference

Feduccia AA, Mithoefer MC. MDMA-assisted psychotherapy for PTSD: are memory reconsolidation and fear extinction underlying mechanisms? *Prog Neuropsychopharmacol Biol Psychiatry* 2018;8(84):221–8.

QUESTION SIX

A 34-year-old woman with PTSD has been treated with exposure therapy, with partial success. Her clinician is considering an adjunct medication. The agent D-cycloserine could be efficacious for reducing symptoms in anxiety disorders because it has been shown to:

A. Modulate glutamate neurotransmission during fear conditioning

B. Modulate glutamate neurotransmission during fear extinction

Anxiety/Stress Disorders and Their Treatment

Answer to Question Six

The correct answer is B.

Choice	Peer answers
Modulate glutamate neurotransmission during fear conditioning	35%
Modulate glutamate neurotransmission during fear extinction	65%

A – Incorrect. When an individual encounters a stressful or fearful experience, the sensory input is relayed to the amygdala, where it is integrated with input from the ventromedial prefrontal cortex (VMPFC) and hippocampus, so that a fear response can be either generated or suppressed. The amygdala may "remember" stimuli associated with that experience by increasing the efficiency of glutamate neurotransmission, so that on future exposure to stimuli, a fear response is more efficiently triggered. If this is not countered by input from the VMPFC to suppress the fear response, fear conditioning proceeds. Because D-cycloserine, as an NMDA co-agonist, may strengthen the efficiency of glutamate neurotransmission, it would theoretically *increase* rather than decrease the likelihood of fear conditioning.

B – Correct. Fear conditioning is not readily reversed, but it can be inhibited through new learning. This new learning is termed fear extinction and is the progressive reduction of the response to a feared stimulus that is repeatedly presented without adverse consequences. Thus, the VMPFC and hippocampus learn a new context for the feared stimulus and send input to the amygdala to suppress the fear response. The "memory" of the conditioned fear is still present, however. Strengthening of synapses involved in fear extinction could help enhance the development of fear extinction learning in the amygdala and reduce symptoms of anxiety disorders. Administration of the D-cycloserine while an individual is receiving exposure therapy could increase the efficiency of glutamate neurotransmission at synapses involved in fear extinction.

Reference

Stahl SM. *Stahl's essential psychopharmacology: the prescriber's guide*, seventh edition. New York, NY: Cambridge University Press; 2020.

QUESTION SEVEN

A 26-year-old patient with panic disorder is ready to begin pharmacotherapy. Which of the following would be appropriate treatment options?

A. Benzodiazepine

B. Selective serotonin reuptake inhibitor (SSRI)

C. A and B

D. Neither A nor B

Anxiety/Stress Disorders and Their Treatment

Answer to Question Seven

The correct answer is C.

Choice	Peer answers
Benzodiazepine	1%
Selective serotonin reuptake inhibitor (SSRI)	35%
A and B	63%
Neither A nor B	1%

A – Partially correct. For panic disorder, benzodiazepines are an appropriate treatment option, although many clinicians prefer not to use them as the first-line option. Benzodiazepines are also appropriate treatment options for generalized anxiety disorder or social anxiety disorder, although again may not be the first-line choice. They do not have evidence of efficacy for PTSD. Most patients with anxiety or stress-related disorders may benefit most from combined treatment with both nonpharmacological options, such as cognitive behavioral therapy, and pharmacological options.

B – Partially correct. SSRIs are appropriate first-line treatment options for panic disorder as well as for generalized anxiety disorder, social anxiety disorder, and PTSD. Most patients with anxiety or stress-related disorders may benefit most from combined treatment with both nonpharmacological options, such as cognitive behavioral therapy, and pharmacological options.

C – Correct. Both benzodiazepines and SSRIs can be used to treat panic disorder, generalized anxiety disorder, and social anxiety disorder.

D – Incorrect.

Reference
Stahl SM. *Stahl's essential psychopharmacology: the prescriber's guide*, seventh edition. New York, NY: Cambridge University Press; 2020.

QUESTION EIGHT

A 4-year-old girl has just been removed from her home by social services due to suspicions of abuse and neglect. Severe early life stress can cause changes in functioning of the hypothalamic–pituitary–adrenal (HPA) axis, which in turn can increase risk for the development of future stress-related disorders. Research suggests that modulation at what level may be necessary in order to prevent the changes in HPA functioning that occur with early stress?

A. Corticotropin-releasing hormone (CRH) gene expression/CRH activity

B. Adrenocorticotropic hormone (ACTH) gene expression/ACTH activity

C. Cortisol gene expression/cortisol activity

Answer to Question Eight

The correct answer is A.

Choice	Peer answers
Corticotropin-releasing hormone (CRH) gene expression/CRH activity	57%
Adrenocorticotropic hormone (ACTH) gene expression/ACTH activity	22%
Cortisol gene expression/cortisol activity	21%

A – Correct. Changes in HPA axis functioning that can occur with severe early life stress may begin with the CRH gene. That is, changes in CRH gene expression precede the other changes that are seen with early mild or severe stress. Thus, in cases of mild stress, it seems that reduced expression of CRH promotes less peptide release in response to stress, and therefore less glucocorticoid release, which ultimately causes upregulation of glucocorticoid receptors. In addition, studies with non-handled rats show that blocking CRH from binding to its type 1 receptor can lead to the same changes and corresponding enhancements in cognitive function. Similarly, blocking CRH1 receptors soon after exposure to early-life chronic stress can normalize hippocampal function in adulthood.

The results of these studies suggest that some of the mechanisms behind the risk for stress-related disorders may be set in motion at a very young age. Accordingly, treatment may need to be administered not after symptoms develop, but rather immediately after – or during – exposure to early life stress, in order to prevent the changes in gene expression that may confer greater risk later in life. This may explain why CRH1 antagonists in major depressive disorder in adults – long after possible exposure to early life stressors – have been mostly ineffective.

B and C – Incorrect.

References

Korosi A, Baram TZ. Plasticity of the stress response early in life: mechanisms and significance. *Dev Psychobiol* 2010;52:661–70.

McClelland S, Korosi A, Cope J, Ivy A, Baram TZ. Emerging roles of epigenetic mechanisms in the enduring effects of early-life stress and experience on learning and memory. *Neurobiol Learning Mem* 2011;96(1):79–88.

Zhou QG, Zhu XH, Nemes AD, Zhu DY. Neuronal nitric oxide synthase and affective disorders. *IBRO Rep* 2018;5:116–32.

QUESTION NINE

A 33-year-old female has had severe symptoms of PTSD, from an assault that occurred 2 years ago. She still experiences flashbacks, nightmares, and an overactive startle response when she is in a context or situation that is similar to where she was when the assault occurred. She may be a candidate for a more novel treatment that combines psychotherapy and pharmacological application of agents (e.g., beta-blockers) to disrupt reconsolidation of her fear memories. This treatment works potentially by:

A. Reactivating the fear memories, making them labile

B. Avoiding or discounting the original fear memories

C. Using a pharmacological agent that blocks protein synthesis associated with the original fear memories

D. Creating new memories to replace the original fear memories

E. A and C

Answer to Question Nine

The correct answer is E.

Choice	Peer answers
Reactivating the fear memories, making them labile	2%
Avoiding or discounting the original fear memories	1%
Using a pharmacological agent that blocks protein synthesis associated with the original fear memories	15%
Creating new memories to replace the original fear memories	6%
A and C	76%

While traumatic memories were once thought to be permanent, recent animal experiments have shown that emotional memories can be weakened or even erased at the time they are re-experienced. The theory of reconsolidation proposes that by re-experiencing a traumatic memory through psychotherapies such as exposure therapy, the memory is reactivated, and can become a labile memory trace. In this labile state, the original fear memory requires protein synthesis for restabilization of the original memory. This offers a window of opportunity to target fear memories with amnestic agents that block protein synthesis. Many animal and human studies have demonstrated that administration of a beta-blocker (e.g., propranolol) prior to or after memory reactivation effectively erased the affective component from the fear memory, without altering the actual recollection of the traumatic event.

A – Partially correct. Reactivating the memory allows it to become destabilized, or labile. This is the first phase of the reconsolidation treatment approach. The erasing of the affective component of the fear memory that has been reported in reconsolidation experiments does not occur if the original fear memory was not first reactivated.

B – Incorrect. The purpose of this treatment approach is to reactivate the original fear memory trace, to allow it to become labile, where protein synthesis can be disrupted.

C – Partially correct. The second component of this treatment approach is to combine the use of a pharmacological agent (e.g., beta-blocker) that has been shown to disrupt protein synthesis for memory consolidation. The noradrenergic beta-blocker propranolol disrupts protein synthesis via the downstream beta-adrenergic receptors/PKA/CREB signaling pathway: one of the molecular cascades that regulate gene transcription required for the consolidation and reconsolidation of memory. The reconsolidation disrupting effects of propranolol were originally demonstrated in animals and later in humans.

D – Incorrect. This treatment approach does not ignore the original fear memory and seek to create new ones about the traumatic event. This approach utilizes exposure to the original traumatic memory, reactivating it and then preventing reconsolidation by blocking protein synthesis, allowing the affective component to be erased.

E – A and C. Correct. Reconsolidation is a two-phase process in which retrieval of a memory initiates a transient period of destabilization, followed by a protein-synthesis-dependent restabilization phase. By reactivating the original memory, and disrupting protein synthesis required for reconsolidation, the affective component can effectively be weakened, or erased.

References

Kindt M, van Emmerick A. New avenues for treating emotional memory disorders: towards a reconsolidation intervention for posttraumatic stress disorder. *Ther Adv Psychopharm* 2016;6(4):283–95.

Stahl SM. *Stahl's essential psychopharmacology*, fifth edition. New York, NY: Cambridge University Press; 2021. (Chapter 8)

Anxiety/Stress Disorders and Their Treatment

QUESTION TEN

Sarah is a 24-year-old patient with generalized anxiety disorder. She is taking a benzodiazepine and has been complaining of sleepiness associated with taking the medication. Which GABA-A alpha subunit has been most associated with sedation properties of benzodiazepines?

A. GABA-A receptors containing alpha-1 subunits

B. GABA-A receptors containing alpha-2 subunits

C. GABA-A receptors containing alpha-3 subunits

D. GABA-A receptors containing alpha-4 subunits

Answer to Question Ten

The correct answer is A.

Choice	Peer answers
GABA-A receptors containing alpha-1 subunits	54%
GABA-A receptors containing alpha-2 subunits	31%
GABA-A receptors containing alpha-3 subunits	11%
GABA-A receptors containing alpha-4 subunits	4%

Currently available benzodiazepines are nonselective for GABA-A receptors with different alpha subunits. Benzodiazepines bind to GABA-A alpha subunits: alpha 1, alpha 2, alpha 3, and alpha 5. Each of these subunits is associated with different effects, and thus benzodiazepines not only cause sedation but are also anxiolytic, cause muscle relaxation, and have alcohol potentiating actions.

A – Correct. Benzodiazepine-sensitive GABA-A receptors with alpha-1 subunits may be most important for regulating sleep and are the presumed targets of numerous sedative-hypnotic agents.

B and C – Incorrect. Benzodiazepine-sensitive GABA-A receptors with alpha-2 subunits and alpha-3 subunits may be most important for regulating anxiety and are the presumed targets of anxiolytic benzodiazepines.

D – Incorrect. GABA-A receptors containing alpha-4 subunits are benzodiazepine-insensitive, are located extrasynaptically, and regulate tonic inhibition.

References

Nuss P. Anxiety disorders and GABA neurotransmission: a disturbance of modulation. *Neuropsychiatr Dis Treat* 2015;11:165–75.

Stahl SM. Selective actions on sleep or anxiety by exploiting GABA-A/benzodiazepine receptor subtypes. *J Clin Psychiatry* 2002;63(3):179–80.

Stahl SM. *Stahl's essential psychopharmacology*, fifth edition. New York, NY: Cambridge University Press; 2021. (Chapter 8)

QUESTION ELEVEN

A man who was severely bitten by a dog as a child is beginning cognitive restructuring therapy to treat his PTSD. He identifies walking down the sidewalk past a person with their dog on a leash as a highly distressing situation, rating his fear during such an encounter as 80/100. He states that he strongly believes any dog is likely to escape its leash and attack him. The next step in cognitive restructuring would be for him to:

A. Put himself in a situation in which he encounters a dog on a leash

B. Identify evidence for and against the thought that the dog would escape and attack him

C. Practice techniques such as breathing exercises while thinking about encountering a dog on a leash

Answer to Question Eleven

The correct answer is B.

Choice	Peer answers
Put himself in a situation in which he encounters a dog on a leash	3%
Identify evidence for and against the thought that the dog would escape and attack him	69%
Practice techniques such as breathing exercises while thinking about encountering a dog on a leash	29%

A – Incorrect. Putting himself in a situation in which he encounters his fear (i.e., a dog) would be part of exposure therapy, but is not part of cognitive restructuring.

B – Correct. Cognitive restructuring is a process by which patients learn to evaluate and modify inaccurate and unhelpful thoughts (e.g., "All dogs are vicious"). There are six main steps of cognitive restructuring: (1) identify a distressing event/thought, (2) identify and rate (0–100) emotions related to the event/thought, (3) identify automatic thoughts associated with the emotions, rate the degree to which one believes them, and select one to challenge, (4) identify evidence in support of and against the thought, (5) generate a response to the thought using the evidence for/against (even though <evidence for>, in fact <evidence against>) and rate the degree of belief in the response, and (6) rerate emotion related to the event/thought.

C – Incorrect. Breathing exercises are not part of cognitive restructuring.

References

Forneris CA, Gartlehner G, Brownley KA et al. Interventions to prevent post-traumatic stress disorder: a systematic review. *Am J Prev Med* 2013;44(6):635–50.

Kliem S, Kroger C. Prevention of chronic PTSD with early cognitive behavioral therapy. A meta-analysis using mixed-effects modeling. *Behav Res Ther* 2013;51(11):753–61.

Stahl SM, Grady MM. *Stahl's illustrated anxiety, stress, and PTSD.* New York, NY: Cambridge University Press; 2010. (Chapter 6)

Zayfert C, Becker CB. *Cognitive-behavioral therapy for PTSD: a case formulation approach.* New York, NY: The Guildford Press; 2007.

QUESTION TWELVE

A 39-year-old veteran presents with comorbid PTSD and substance abuse. Her care provider recommends addressing her PTSD and substance use disorder (SUD) simultaneously. Which of the following statements is true regarding managing co-occurring PTSD and SUD?

A. Individualized trauma-focused PTSD treatment, such as Prolonged Exposure, alongside SUD intervention can reduce PTSD severity and drug/alcohol use

B. Non-trauma-focused PTSD therapies, such as Seeking Safety, are more effective than treatment as usual for reducing PTSD symptoms in patients with PTSD and SUD

C. The presence of an SUD should prevent concurrent treatment and SUD must be stabilized prior to treating the PTSD

Answer to Question Twelve

The correct answer is A.

Choice	Peer answers
Individualized trauma-focused PTSD treatment, such as Prolonged Exposure, alongside SUD intervention can reduce PTSD severity and drug/alcohol use	68%
Non-trauma-focused PTSD therapies, such as Seeking Safety, are more effective than treatment as usual for reducing PTSD symptoms in patients with PTSD and SUD	17%
The presence of an SUD should prevent concurrent treatment and SUD must be stabilized prior to treating the PTSD	16%

A – Correct. Individual trauma-focused PTSD therapies that have a primary component of exposure and/or cognitive restructuring, such as Prolonged Exposure, when delivered together with SUD interventions, were more likely than SUD treatment alone or treatment as usual to improve PTSD symptoms in individuals with co-occurring PTSD and SUD. Patients with PTSD and SUD can tolerate and benefit from evidence-based trauma-focused PTSD treatment such as Prolonged Exposure.

B – Incorrect. Non-trauma-focused PTSD therapies (e.g., Seeking Safety), when delivered together with an SUD therapy, do not improve PTSD symptoms in individuals with SUDs more than SUD treatment alone or treatment as usual. Non-trauma-focused therapies such as Seeking Safety for the treatment of PTSD in the context of co-occurring SUD are not recommended.

C – Incorrect. Recent research has shown that patients with PTSD and SUD (including nicotine use disorder) can both tolerate and benefit from concurrent treatment for both conditions, even in the most severe cases.

References

Management of Posttraumatic Stress Disorder Work Group. VA/DOD Clinical practice guideline: management of posttraumatic stress disorder and acute stress reaction 2017. Washington DC; 2017.

Roberts NP, Roberts PA, Jones N, Bisson JI. Psychological interventions for post-traumatic stress disorder and comorbid substance use disorder: a systematic review and meta-analysis. *Clin Psychol Rev* 2015;38:25–38.

Stahl SM, Grady MM. *Stahl's illustrated anxiety, stress, and PTSD*. New York, NY: Cambridge University Press; 2010. (Chapter 6)

Zandberg LJ, Rosenfield D, McLean CP et al. Concurrent treatment of posttraumatic stress disorder and alcohol dependence: predictors and moderators of outcome. *J Consult Clin Psychol* 2016;84(1):43–56.

Anxiety/Stress Disorders and Their Treatment

QUESTION THIRTEEN

Which of the following drugs can diminish anxiety but does NOT have sedative, hypnotic, anticonvulsant, or musculoskeletal relaxing activity?

A. Buspirone

B. Diazepam

C. Haloperidol

D. Mirtazapine

Anxiety/Stress Disorders and Their Treatment

Answer to Question Thirteen

The correct answer is A.

Choice	Peer answers
Buspirone	97%
Diazepam	0%
Haloperidol	1%
Mirtazapine	1%

A – Correct. Buspirone is a serotonin 5HT1A receptor partial agonist used to treat anxiety. Buspirone's partial agonist actions at presynaptic somatodendritic serotonin autoreceptors may theoretically enhance serotonergic activity and contribute to antidepressant actions. The partial agonist actions postsynaptically may theoretically diminish serotonergic activity and contribute to anxiolytic actions. It does not produce significant sedation, hypnotic, anticonvulsant, or musculoskeletal relaxing effects.

B – Incorrect. Diazepam is a benzodiazepine that is nonspecific and works by binding to multiple GABA-A receptor subtypes, including the alpha-1 subunit that is important for sedation.

C – Incorrect. By blocking dopamine 2 receptors in the striatum, haloperidol can cause motor side effects. Also, by blocking alpha 1 adrenergic receptors, it can cause dizziness, sedation, and hypotension.

D – Incorrect. Mirtazapine blocks 5HT2A, 5HT2C, and 5HT3 serotonin receptors and blocks H1 histamine receptors. Histamine 1 receptor antagonism may explain sedative effects.

References

Piszczek L, Piszczek A, Kuczmanska J, Audero E, Gross CT. Modulation of anxiety by cortical serotonin 1A receptors. *Front Behav Neurosci* 2015;9:48.

Stahl SM. *Stahl's essential psychopharmacology: the prescriber's guide*, seventh edition. New York, NY: Cambridge University Press; 2020.

Stahl SM. *Stahl's essential psychopharmacology*, fifth edition. New York, NY: Cambridge University Press; 2021. (Chapter 8)

QUESTION FOURTEEN

A 38-year-old man with a history of treatment-resistant PTSD has now experienced improvement on quetiapine 300 mg/day, duloxetine 90 mg/day, and zolpidem 10 mg at bedtime. However, he complains of ongoing nightmares and difficulty staying asleep. He was previously initiated on prazosin 3 mg at bedtime, but he experienced intolerable dizziness, and it was discontinued. Can this patient be rechallenged with prazosin? If so, at what dose?

A. Yes; dose should be initiated at 1 mg at bedtime

B. Yes; dose should be initiated at 3 mg at bedtime

C. No; prazosin is contraindicated with quetiapine

D. No; prazosin should not be reattempted in patients with previous intolerability

Answer to Question Fourteen

The correct answer is A.

Choice	Peer answers
Yes; dose should be initiated at 1 mg at bedtime	93%
Yes; dose should be initiated at 3 mg at bedtime	1%
No; prazosin is contraindicated with quetiapine	3%
No; prazosin should not be reattempted in patients with previous intolerability	4%

A – Correct. Prazosin, an alpha 1 antagonist, can be an effective treatment for nightmares in PTSD. The initial dose of prazosin should be 1 mg at bedtime and titrated up 1 mg every 2–3 days to decrease the risk of syncope.

B – Incorrect. There is risk of "first-dose effect" syncope with sudden loss of consciousness (1%) with an initial dose of at least 2 mg; thus, 3 mg would be too high for an initiation dose.

C – Incorrect. Prazosin is not contraindicated with quetiapine. The only contraindications for prazosin are proven allergy to prazosin or to quinazolines (e.g., the cancer medications gefitinib and erlotinib or the prostatic hyperplasia medications alfuzosin and bunazosin).

D – Incorrect. There is no reason why a patient cannot be rechallenged with prazosin if they experienced previous intolerability (assuming they did not have an allergic reaction). Patients may require slower titration or lower dose if they have previously not tolerated prazosin.

References

Kung A, Espinel Z, Lalpid MI. Treatment of nightmares with prazosin: a systematic review. *Mayo Clin Proc* 2012;87(9):890–900.

Simon PY, Rousseau PF. Treatment of post-traumatic stress disorders with the alpha-1 adrenergic antagonist prazosin. *Can J Psychiatry* 2017;62(3):186–98.

Stahl SM. *Stahl's essential psychopharmacology: the prescriber's guide*, seventh edition. New York, NY: Cambridge University Press; 2020.

QUESTION FIFTEEN

A 28-year-old combat veteran with PTSD has not responded to multiple trials of oral medication. He suffers from nightmares, rarely maintains sleep longer than 2 hours, and has lost interest in his family life, which is particularly difficult for his wife given that she is pregnant with their first child. The role of glutamate in traumatic memory formation and extinction suggests that ketamine may be beneficial; however, the potential side effect profile of ketamine could also be concerning for patients with PTSD. In a recent controlled proof-of-concept study in PTSD, ketamine:

A. Did not reduce PTSD symptoms and caused transient worsening of dissociative symptoms

B. Did not reduce PTSD symptoms and caused sustained worsening of dissociative symptoms

C. Reduced PTSD symptoms and caused transient worsening of dissociative symptoms

D. Reduced PTSD symptoms and caused sustained worsening of dissociative symptoms

Anxiety/Stress Disorders and Their Treatment

Answer to Question Fifteen

The correct answer is C.

Choice	Peer answers
Did not reduce PTSD symptoms and caused transient worsening of dissociative symptoms	9%
Did not reduce PTSD symptoms and caused sustained worsening of dissociative symptoms	3%
Reduced PTSD symptoms and caused transient worsening of dissociative symptoms	83%
Reduced PTSD symptoms and caused sustained worsening of dissociative symptoms	4%

Like D-cycloserine, ketamine could theoretically strengthen the efficiency of glutamate neurotransmission at synapses involved in fear extinction and thus improve symptoms of PTSD. In a proof-of-concept, double-blind, randomized, crossover trial comparing ketamine to the active placebo control midazolam, researchers found that ketamine infusion was associated with significant reduction in PTSD symptom severity, assessed 24 hours after infusion. This remained significant after adjusting for depressive symptom severity. In the study, ketamine caused transient worsening of dissociative symptoms, but this was not sustained. The clinical relevance of this study will be subject both to successful replication and to identification of an alternate method of ketamine administration. Methods that are under investigation for depression include intranasal and intramuscular.

A – Incorrect. It is true that ketamine caused transient worsening of dissociative symptoms; however, it also reduced PTSD symptoms.

B – Incorrect. Ketamine caused transient but not sustained worsening of dissociative symptoms.

C – Correct. Ketamine reduced PTSD symptoms and caused transient worsening of dissociative symptoms.

D – Incorrect. Ketamine reduced PTSD symptoms but did not cause sustained worsening of dissociative symptoms.

References

Feder A, Parides MK, Murrough JW et al. Efficacy of intravenous ketamine for treatment of chronic posttraumatic stress disorder: a randomized clinical trial. *JAMA Psychiatry* 2014;71(6):681–8.

Womble AL. Effects of ketamine on major depressive disorder in a patient with posttraumatic stress disorder. *AANA J* 2013;81(2):118–19.

CHAPTER PEER COMPARISON

For the Anxiety/Stress Disorders section, the correct answer was selected 74% of the time.

Anxiety/Stress Disorders and Their Treatment

3   BASIC NEUROSCIENCE AND PHARMACOLOGICAL CONCEPTS

QUESTION ONE

An excitatory signal is received at the dendrite of a pyramidal glutamate neuron. When the signal is released from the incoming presynaptic dopaminergic axon, it is received as an inhibitory signal. However, this signal is not integrated properly with other incoming signals to that neuron. Which is the most likely site at which the error of integrating this signal with other incoming signals occurred?

A. Dendritic membrane

B. Soma

C. Axonal zone

D. Presynaptic zone

Answer to Question One

The correct answer is B.

Choice	Peer answers
Dendritic membrane	16%
Soma	47%
Axonal zone	10%
Presynaptic zone	26%

A – Incorrect. Dendritic membrane is the site of signal detection; signal integration does not occur here.

B – Correct. Soma is the site that integrates chemical encoding of signal transduction from all incoming signals; improper signal integration is most likely at this site.

C – Incorrect. Axonal zone is the site of signal propagation; signal integration does not occur here.

D – Incorrect. Presynaptic zone is the site of signal output; signal integration does not occur here.

Reference

Stahl SM. *Stahl's essential psychopharmacology*, fifth edition. New York, NY: Cambridge University Press; 2021. (Chapter 1)

QUESTION TWO

Which brain imaging technique used in psychiatry research provides measurements of both structure and function of the human brain?

A. Electroencephalography

B. Magnetic resonance imaging

C. Positron emission tomography

D. Transcranial magnetic stimulation

Basic Neuroscience and Pharmacological Concepts

Answer to Question Two

The correct answer is B.

Choice	Peer answers
Electroencephalography	5%
Magnetic resonance imaging	61%
Positron emission tomography	33%
Transcranial magnetic stimulation	2%

A – Incorrect. Electroencephalography, or EEG, may be used to identify electrical activity in the brain. Electrodes placed around the scalp provide a general location of electrical activity; however, EEG does not provide measurements of brain structure.

B – Correct. Magnetic resonance imaging, or MRI, may be used to measure brain structure and function. Structural MRI (sMRI) and diffusion tensor imaging (DTI) are types of MRI acquisitions that can be used to obtain structural measurements of the brain. Functional MRI (fMRI) is a type of MRI acquisition that measures brain activity by way of the blood-oxygen-level-dependent (BOLD) signal.

C – Incorrect. Positron emission tomography, or PET, may be used to identify chemical activity, which is a measure of brain function; however, it is not used to provide measurements of brain structure. PET may be combined with MRI or computerized tomography to make more specific conclusions about the structural location of chemical activity in the brain.

D – Incorrect. Transcranial magnetic stimulation, or TMS, is not a neuroimaging technique. TMS is used to stimulate nerve cells in the brain and the resultant motor output may provide indirect information on brain function.

Reference

Power BD, Nguyen T, Hayhow B, Looi JCL. Neuroimaging in psychiatry: an update on neuroimaging in the clinical setting. *Australas Psychiatry* 2016;24(2):157–63.

QUESTION THREE

Which of the following are involved in regulating neurotransmission via excitation–secretion coupling?

A. Voltage-sensitive sodium channels

B. Voltage-sensitive calcium channels

C. Both A and B

D. Neither A nor B

Answer to Question Three

The correct answer is C.

Choice	Peer answers
Voltage-sensitive sodium channels	8%
Voltage-sensitive calcium channels	8%
Both A and B	82%
Neither A nor B	2%

A – Partially correct.

B – Partially correct.

C – Correct. Propagation of an action potential to the axon terminal is mediated by voltage-sensitive sodium channels. Influx of sodium through voltage-sensitive sodium channels at the axon terminal leads to opening of voltage-sensitive calcium channels, also at the axon terminal. Influx of calcium through the open voltage-sensitive calcium channels leads to docking of synaptic vesicles and secretion of neurotransmitter into the synapse.

D – Incorrect.

Reference
Stahl SM. *Stahl's essential psychopharmacology*, fifth edition. New York, NY: Cambridge University Press; 2021. (Chapter 3)

QUESTION FOUR

Agonists cause ligand-gated ion channels to:

A. Open wider

B. Open for longer duration of time

C. Open more frequently

D. A and B

E. A and C

Basic Neuroscience and Pharmacological Concepts

Answer to Question Four

The correct answer is C.

Choice	Peer answers
Open wider	2%
Open for longer duration of time	10%
Open more frequently	43%
A and B	31%
A and C	14%

A – Incorrect. Agonists do not cause ligand-gated receptors to open wider.

B – Incorrect. Agonists do not cause ligand-gated receptors to open for longer durations of time.

C – Correct. Agonists cause ligand-gated ion channels to open more frequently.

D – Incorrect.

E – Incorrect.

Reference

Stahl SM. *Stahl's essential psychopharmacology*, fifth edition. New York, NY: Cambridge University Press; 2021. (Chapter 3)

QUESTION FIVE

Presynaptic reuptake transporters are a major method of inactivation for which of the following?

A. Serotonin

B. Serotonin and gamma-aminobutyric acid (GABA)

C. Serotonin, GABA, and histamine

D. Serotonin, GABA, histamine, and neuropeptides

Basic Neuroscience and Pharmacological Concepts

Answer to Question Five

The correct answer is B.

Choice	Peer answers
Serotonin	27%
Serotonin and gamma-aminobutyric acid (GABA)	50%
Serotonin, GABA, and histamine	12%
Serotonin, GABA, histamine, and neuropeptides	12%

A – Partially correct.

B – Correct. Both monoamines such as serotonin and amino acid neurotransmitters such as GABA are inactivated primarily via presynaptic transporters.

C – Incorrect. Histamine does not have a known presynaptic reuptake transporter and is instead inactivated via enzymatic degradation.

D – Incorrect. Histamine and neuropeptides do not have known presynaptic reuptake transporters. Histamine is inactivated enzymatically, and neuropeptides are inactivated by diffusion, sequestration, and enzymatic destruction.

Reference

Stahl SM. *Stahl's essential psychopharmacology*, fifth edition. New York, NY: Cambridge University Press; 2021. (Chapter 2)

QUESTION SIX

A neuron is infected with a toxin and causes a rather sudden inflammatory reaction. You detect a high concentration of cytokines in the surrounding area. Which process has taken place?

A. Apoptosis

B. Excitotoxicity

C. Necrosis

D. Neurogenesis

E. Synaptogenesis

Basic Neuroscience and Pharmacological Concepts

Answer to Question Six

The correct answer is C.

Choice	Peer answers
Apoptosis	30%
Excitotoxicity	22%
Necrosis	45%
Neurogenesis	2%
Synaptogenesis	1%

A – Incorrect. Apoptosis is triggered by a cell's own genetic machinery, causing the cell to just "fade away." The more caustic inflammatory response from cell death is associated with the neural selection process of necrosis. Cells that commit suicide (apoptosis) die in a more benign manner than when they are the victims of homicide (necrosis).

B – Incorrect. Excitotoxicity is a process of synaptic damage from "over-excitation," excessive amounts of which can result in cell death.

C – Correct. Necrosis is the neural selection process in which a cell is poisoned, suffocated, or otherwise destroyed by a toxin after which the cell explodes and causes an inflammatory reaction.

D – Incorrect. Neurogenesis is the process of forming neurons.

E – Incorrect. Synaptogenesis is the process of forming synapses.

Reference

Stahl SM. *Stahl's essential psychopharmacology*, fifth edition. New York, NY: Cambridge University Press; 2021. (Chapter 1)

QUESTION SEVEN

Communication between human central nervous system neurons at synapses is:

A. Chemical

B. Electrical

C. Both A and B

D. Neither A nor B

Basic Neuroscience and Pharmacological Concepts

Answer to Question Seven

The correct answer is A.

Choice	Peer answers
Chemical	53%
Electrical	2%
Both A and B	45%
Neither A nor B	0%

A – Correct. The communication between neurons at synapses is mediated by neurotransmitter molecules and is therefore chemical.

B – Incorrect. Although electrical communication occurs within neurons during the propagation of an action potential, communication at synapses is chemical.

C – Incorrect.

D – Incorrect.

Reference

Stahl SM. *Stahl's essential psychopharmacology*, fifth edition. New York, NY: Cambridge University Press; 2021. (Chapter 1)

QUESTION EIGHT

A serotonin molecule binds to a 5HT2A receptor causing electrical impulses to be sent down a GABA neuron's axon terminal, eventually releasing GABA to the GABA-A receptor of its postsynaptic neuron. Which type of neurotransmission does this describe?

A. Classic synaptic neurotransmission

B. Retrograde neurotransmission

C. Volume neurotransmission

D. Signal transduction cascade

Answer to Question Eight

The correct answer is A.

Choice	Peer answers
Classic synaptic neurotransmission	71%
Retrograde neurotransmission	5%
Volume neurotransmission	1%
Signal transduction cascade	23%

A – Correct. Classic synaptic neurotransmission is the most common and well-known process of neurotransmission. It involves the anterograde transduction of a chemical signal to electrical impulses and back to chemical signals for the next neuron.

B – Incorrect. Retrograde neurotransmission is the "reverse" neurotransmission process in which a postsynaptic neuron communicates with a presynaptic neuron.

C – Incorrect. Volume neurotransmission is the process of neurotransmission without a synapse, which is also called nonsynaptic diffusion.

D – Incorrect. Signal transduction cascade is the larger process of neurocommunication that involves long strings of chemical and ionic signals.

Reference

Stahl SM. *Stahl's essential psychopharmacology*, fifth edition. New York, NY: Cambridge University Press; 2021. (Chapter 1)

QUESTION NINE

A receptor with four transmembrane regions changes conformation as GABA binds. Which system is this process describing?

A. Ligand-gated ion channel

B. Presynaptic transporter

C. Voltage-sensitive ion channel

Answer to Question Nine

The correct answer is A.

Choice	Peer answers
Ligand-gated ion channel	85%
Presynaptic transporter	7%
Voltage-sensitive ion channel	8%

A – Correct. Ligand-gated ion channels are four-transmembrane region ion channels that open and close under instruction from bound neurotransmitters.

B – Incorrect. Presynaptic transporters are twelve-transmembrane region transporters that bind to neurotransmitters to transport them across the presynaptic membrane.

C – Incorrect. Voltage-sensitive ion channels are six-transmembrane region ion channels that open and close under instruction from charges or voltages as determined by ion flow.

Reference

Stahl SM. *Stahl's essential psychopharmacology*, fifth edition. New York, NY: Cambridge University Press; 2021. (Chapters 2, 3)

QUESTION TEN

The direct role of transcription factors is to:

A. Cause neurotransmitter release

B. Influence gene expression

C. Synthesize enzymes

D. Trigger signal transduction cascades

Answer to Question Ten

The correct answer is B.

Choice	Peer answers
Cause neurotransmitter release	3%
Influence gene expression	81%
Synthesize enzymes	9%
Trigger signal transduction cascades	6%

A – Incorrect. Transcription factors do not directly cause neurotransmitter release.

B – Correct. Transcription factors are proteins that bind to promoter sequences of DNA to turn gene expression on and off.

C – Incorrect. Transcription factors do not directly cause enzyme synthesis.

D – Incorrect. Transcription factors do not directly trigger signal transduction cascades.

Reference
Stahl SM. *Stahl's essential psychopharmacology*, fifth edition. New York, NY: Cambridge University Press; 2021. (Chapter 1)

QUESTION ELEVEN

Which of the following is the most likely impetus for upregulation of D2 receptors on a striatal dopamine neuron?

A. A bound receptor is taken out of circulation

B. A new receptor is bound and put to use

C. A D2 agonist persistently binds to the receptor

D. A D2 antagonist persistently binds to the receptor

Answer to Question Eleven

The correct answer is D.

Choice	Peer answers
A bound receptor is taken out of circulation	3%
A new receptor is bound and put to use	4%
A D2 agonist persistently binds to the receptor	28%
A D2 antagonist persistently binds to the receptor	65%

A – Incorrect. A bound receptor is usually taken out of circulation when the neuron wants to decrease, not increase, the number of receptors.

B – Incorrect. A new receptor being bound and put to use is a result, not an impetus, of upregulation.

C – Incorrect. Agonists can mimic neurotransmitter actions, potentially signaling the neuron to downregulate synthesis of that receptor type.

D – Correct. Antagonists can oppose neurotransmitter actions, potentially signaling the neuron to upregulate synthesis of that receptor type.

Reference

Stahl SM. *Stahl's essential psychopharmacology*, fifth edition. New York, NY: Cambridge University Press; 2021. (Chapters 3, 5)

QUESTION TWELVE

What is the correct order and direction of ion flow into and out of a neuron experiencing an action potential?

A. Na^+ in, K^+ out, Ca^{2+} in

B. Ca^{2+} in, K^+ out, Na^+ in

C. K^+ in, Na^+ in, Ca^{2+} in

D. Na^+ in, Ca^{2+} in, K^+ out

E. Ca^{2+} in, Na^+ out, K^+ out

F. K^+ in, Ca^{2+} in, Na^+ out

Answer to Question Twelve

The correct answer is D.

Choice	Peer answers
Na^+ in, K^+ out, Ca^{2+} in	35%
Ca^{2+} in, K^+ out, Na^+ in	3%
K^+ in, Na^+ in, Ca^{2+} in	3%
Na^+ in, Ca^{2+} in, K^+ out	53%
Ca^{2+} in, Na^+ out, K^+ out	3%
K^+ in, Ca^{2+} in, Na^+ out	3%

A, B, C, E, and F – Incorrect.

D – Correct. Sodium enters the cell followed by an influx of calcium; potassium exits the neuron at the end of the action potential, restoring the baseline electrical charge in the cell.

Reference

Stahl SM. *Stahl's essential psychopharmacology*, fifth edition. New York, NY: Cambridge University Press; 2021. (Chapter 3)

QUESTION THIRTEEN

What are the molecular mechanisms of epigenetics?

A. Molecular gates are opened by acetylation and/or demethylation of histones, allowing transcription factors access to genes, thus activating them

B. Molecular gates are opened by deacetylation and/or methylation of histones, allowing transcription factors access to genes, thus activating them

C. Molecular gates are closed by deacetylation and/or methylation of histones, preventing access of transcription factors to genes, thus silencing them

D. A and C

Basic Neuroscience and Pharmacological Concepts

Answer to Question Thirteen

The correct answer is D.

Choice	Peer answers
Molecular gates are opened by acetylation and/or demethylation of histones, allowing transcription factors access to genes, thus activating them	12%
Molecular gates are opened by deacetylation and/or methylation of histones, allowing transcription factors access to genes, thus activating them	11%
Molecular gates are closed by deacetylation and/or methylation of histones, preventing access of transcription factors to genes, thus silencing them	3%
A and C	74%

A – Partially correct. Epigenetics is a process that determines whether a given gene is expressed or silenced. Epigenetic control over whether genes are activated (i.e., expressed) or silenced is achieved by the modification of chromatin. Acetylation and demethylation of histones decompress the chromatin, opening the molecular gates, allowing transcription factors to get to the promoter regions of genes and activate them.

B – Incorrect.

C – Partially correct. Methylation of histones can silence genes, whereas demethylation of histones can activate genes. Methylation of DNA can result in deacetylation of histones by activating enzymes called histone deacetylases (HDACs). Deacetylation of histones also has a silencing effect on gene expression. Methylation and deacetylation compress chromatin, closing the molecular gates, which prevents the transcription factors from accessing the promoter regions that activate genes, thus silencing them.

D – Correct.

Reference

Stahl SM. *Stahl's essential psychopharmacology*, fifth edition. New York, NY: Cambridge University Press; 2021. (Chapter 1)

QUESTION FOURTEEN

N-methyl-D-aspartate (NMDA) receptors are activated by:

A. Glutamate

B. Glycine

C. Depolarization

D. Glutamate and glycine

E. Glutamate and depolarization

F. Glycine and depolarization

G. Glutamate, glycine, and depolarization

Answer to Question Fourteen

The correct answer is G.

Choice	Peer answers
Glutamate	17%
Glycine	0%
Depolarization	0%
Glutamate and glycine	17%
Glutamate and depolarization	15%
Glycine and depolarization	1%
Glutamate, glycine, and depolarization	48%

A, B, C, D, E, and F – Incorrect.

G – Correct. NMDA receptors are ligand-gated ion channels that regulate excitatory postsynaptic neurotransmission triggered by glutamate. In the resting state, NMDA receptors are blocked by magnesium, which plugs the calcium channel. Opening of NMDA glutamate receptors requires the presence of both glutamate and glycine, each of which bind to a different site on the receptor. When magnesium is also bound and the membrane is not depolarized, it prevents the effects of glutamate and glycine and thus does not allow the ion channel to open. In order for the channel to open and permit calcium entry, depolarization must remove magnesium while both glutamate and glycine are bound to their sites.

Reference

Stahl SM. *Stahl's essential psychopharmacology*, fifth edition. New York, NY: Cambridge University Press; 2021. (Chapter 2)

QUESTION FIFTEEN

Neurogenesis occurs in adults:

A. Only in the dentate gyrus of the hippocampus

B. In the dentate gyrus of the hippocampus and in the olfactory bulb

C. In the dentate gyrus of the hippocampus, in the olfactory bulb, and in the lateral nucleus of the amygdala

D. Throughout the brain

Basic Neuroscience and Pharmacological Concepts

Answer to Question Fifteen

The correct answer is B.

Choice	Peer answers
Only in the dentate gyrus of the hippocampus	7%
In the dentate gyrus of the hippocampus and in the olfactory bulb	37%
In the dentate gyrus of the hippocampus, in the olfactory bulb, and in the lateral nucleus of the amygdala	19%
Throughout the brain	38%

A – Partially correct. Although adult neurogenesis does occur in the dentate gyrus, this is not the only brain region where adult neurogenesis occurs.

B – Correct. Adult neurogenesis occurs in both the dentate gyrus of the hippocampus and in the olfactory bulb.

C – Incorrect. Although adult neurogenesis occurs in both the dentate gyrus and the olfactory bulb, there is no evidence that adult neurogenesis occurs in the lateral nucleus of the amygdala.

D – Incorrect. Adult neurogenesis occurs only in the dentate gyrus and in the olfactory bulb.

References

Hagg T. Molecular regulation of adult CNS neurogenesis: an integrated view. *Trends Neurosci* 2005;28(11):589–95.

Ming GL, Song H. Adult neurogenesis in the mammalian brain: significant answers and significant questions. *Neuron* 2011;70(4):687–702.

QUESTION SIXTEEN

A signal transduction cascade passes its message from an extracellular first messenger to an intracellular second messenger. In the case of the G-protein-linked systems, the second messenger is a:

A. Chemical

B. Hormone

C. Ion

D. Kinase enzyme

Answer to Question Sixteen

The correct answer is A.

Choice	Peer answers
Chemical	50%
Hormone	10%
Ion	13%
Kinase enzyme	27%

A – Correct. For a G-protein-linked system the second messenger is a chemical. The four key elements to the G-protein second-messenger system are: (1) the first messenger neurotransmitter; (2) a receptor for the neurotransmitter that belongs to the receptor superfamily in which all have the structure of seven transmembrane regions; (3) a G-protein capable of binding both to certain conformations of the neurotransmitter receptor and to the enzyme system that can synthesize the second messenger; (4) the enzyme system itself for the second messenger.

B – Incorrect. For some hormone-linked systems, a second messenger is formed when a hormone finds its receptor in the cytoplasm and binds to it to form a hormone–nuclear receptor complex. For a G-protein-linked system the second messenger is a chemical.

C – Incorrect. For an ion-channel-linked system, the second messenger can be an ion, such as calcium. For a G-protein-linked system the second messenger is a chemical.

D – Incorrect. For neurotrophins, a complex set of second messengers exist, including proteins that are kinase enzymes. For a G-protein-linked system the second messenger is a chemical.

Reference
Stahl SM. *Stahl's essential psychopharmacology*, fifth edition. New York, NY: Cambridge University Press; 2021. (Chapter 1)

CHAPTER PEER COMPARISON

For the Basic Neuroscience section, the correct answer was selected 59% of the time.

4 BIPOLAR DISORDER AND ITS TREATMENT

QUESTION ONE

A 25-year-old woman has recently been diagnosed with bipolar disorder, 6 years after her symptoms began. She has had no mood stabilizing treatment in that time. According to the kindling model and allostatic load hypothesis, what progressive pattern of illness would you expect this patient to have exhibited over the course of the last 6 years?

A. Shorter interval between episodes, worsened emotionality, worsened cognitive impairment

B. Longer interval between episodes, worsened emotionality, worsened cognitive impairment

C. Shorter interval between episodes, worsened emotionality, minimal change in cognitive impairment

D. Longer interval between episodes, worsened emotionality, minimal change in cognitive impairment

Answer to Question One

The correct answer is A.

Choice	Peer answers
Shorter interval between episodes, worsened emotionality, worsened cognitive impairment	77%
Longer interval between episodes, worsened emotionality, worsened cognitive impairment	4%
Shorter interval between episodes, worsened emotionality, minimal change in cognitive impairment	15%
Longer interval between episodes, worsened emotionality, minimal change in cognitive impairment	4%

A – Correct. Throughout the course of illness, patients with bipolar disorder will experience manic or hypomanic episodes, depressive episodes, and inter-episode periods during which they are generally well but may have subsyndromal symptoms. The pattern of episodes can differ for each patient; however, in general the clinical course of bipolar disorder is progressive. That is, as the number of episodes a person has had increases, the **interval between episodes gets shorter** and **emotionality may worsen**. In addition, **cognitive impairment seems to worsen** with the length of illness. Increasing episode number is also associated with reduced likelihood of treatment response.

Models for how these changes may come to be posit that recurrent mood episodes are associated with repeated physiological insults that add up and kindle, like a spark bursting into fire. This could compromise endogenous compensatory mechanisms, leading to cell apoptosis that in turn causes rewiring of the brain circuits involved in mood regulation and cognition. This can render one more vulnerable to the effects of stressors, increasing risk of future episodes and thus perpetuating the vicious spiral.

B, C, and D – Incorrect.

References

Berk M, **Kapczinski F**, **Andreazza AC** et al. Pathways underlying neuroprogression in bipolar disorder: focus on inflammation, oxidative stress, and neurotrophic factors. *Neurosci Biobehav Rev* 2011;35(3):804–17.

Bipolar Disorder and Its Treatment

Berk M, Post R, Ratheesh A et al. Staging in bipolar disorder: from theoretical framework to clinical utility. *World Psychiatry* 2017;16(3):236–44.

Kapczinski F, Vieta E, Andreazza AC et al. Allostatic load in bipolar disorder: implications for pathophysiology and treatment. *Neurosci Biobehav Rev* 2008;32:675–92.

Post RM. Kindling and sensitization as models for affective episode recurrence, cyclicity, and tolerance phenomena. *Neurosci Biobehav Rev* 2007;31:858–73.

Bipolar Disorder and Its Treatment

QUESTION TWO

A 32-year-old woman with bipolar I disorder has just found out that she is 6 weeks pregnant. Her mania has been stable on a combination of lithium, valproate, and quetiapine, but she is unsure about the safety of maintaining her medications during her pregnancy. Which, if any, of the patient's medications has known teratogenic effects?

A. Lithium

B. Valproate

C. Quetiapine

D. A and B

E. A, B, and C

Answer to Question Two

The correct answer is D.

Choice	Peer answers
Lithium	2%
Valproate	12%
Quetiapine	1%
A and B	79%
A, B, and C	6%

A – Partially correct. Lithium has evidence of increased risk of major birth defects and cardiac anomalies, especially Ebstein's anomaly, although a recent review suggested that the risk of cardiac anomalies may be overemphasized. With lithium, the risk of Ebstein's anomaly is perhaps 1/2500 (basal risk is 1/20 000). It is typically detectable in utero by ultrasonography and can often be corrected surgically after birth. No long-term neurobehavioral effects of late-term neonatal lithium exposure have been observed. Lithium is not contraindicated during pregnancy, and the risks must be weighed against the benefits. If lithium is continued, serum lithium levels must be monitored every 4 weeks, then every week beginning at 36 weeks. Lithium administration during delivery may be associated with hypotonia in the infant, and most recommend withholding lithium for 24–48 hours before delivery, with monitoring during and after delivery of both baby and mother.

B – Partially correct. Valproate is associated with increased risk of neural tube defects (e.g., spina bifida) and other congenital anomalies. Cases of developmental delay in the absence of teratogenicity associated with fetal exposure have also been identified. Increased risk of lower cognitive test scores in children whose mothers took valproate during pregnancy has also been observed. Generally, it is recommended to discontinue valproate during pregnancy. If valproate is continued, clotting parameters should be monitored and tests to detect birth defects should be performed. Patients should begin folate 1 mg/day early in pregnancy to reduce risk of neural tube defects and consider vitamin K during the last 6 weeks of pregnancy to reduce risks of bleeding.

C – Incorrect. Quetiapine does not have known teratogenic effects, and cumulative data with atypical antipsychotics do not show a risk of major malformations. There is a risk of abnormal muscle movements and withdrawal symptoms in newborns whose mothers took an antipsychotic during the third trimester; symptoms may include agitation, abnormally increased or decreased muscle tone, tremor, sleepiness, severe difficulty breathing, and difficulty feeding. If quetiapine or another atypical antipsychotic is used during pregnancy, weight gain and the risk for gestational diabetes should be more carefully monitored, with glucose tolerance testing (as opposed to glucose challenge testing) at 14–16 weeks and again at 28 weeks. After delivery, infants should be monitored for neonatal withdrawal, toxicity, extrapyramidal side effects, and sedation.

D – Correct. Lithium and valproate both have known teratogenic effects.

E – Incorrect.

References

Galbally M, Snellen M, Power J. Antipsychotic drugs in pregnancy: a review of their maternal and fetal effects. *Ther Adv Drug Saf* 2014;5(2):100–9.

Stahl SM. *Stahl's essential psychopharmacology: the prescriber's guide*, seventh edition. New York, NY: Cambridge University Press; 2020.

Yacobi S, Ornoy A. Is lithium a real teratogen? What can we conclude from the prospective versus retrospective studies? A review. *Isr J Psychiatry Relat Sci* 2008;45(2):95–106.

Bipolar Disorder and Its Treatment

QUESTION THREE

A 25-year-old woman presents with a major depressive episode. She has a history of hospitalizations and treatment for manic episodes but is not currently taking any medication. The agents with the strongest evidence of efficacy in bipolar depression are:

A. Lamotrigine, lithium, quetiapine

B. Quetiapine, olanzapine-fluoxetine, lurasidone

C. Olanzapine-fluoxetine, lurasidone, lamotrigine

D. Lurasidone, lamotrigine, lithium

Bipolar Disorder and Its Treatment

Answer to Question Three

The correct answer is B.

Choice	Peer answers
Lamotrigine, lithium, quetiapine	20%
Quetiapine, olanzapine-fluoxetine, lurasidone	51%
Olanzapine-fluoxetine, lurasidone, lamotrigine	14%
Lurasidone, lamotrigine, lithium	15%

A – Incorrect. Controlled data assessing the efficacy of lithium in bipolar depression are limited; in a recent network meta-analysis lithium was not found to be effective compared to placebo in acute bipolar depression. However, lithium does have evidence for reducing suicidality. In the same network meta-analysis, lamotrigine was effective compared to placebo in terms of response but not remission.

B – Correct. Quetiapine, olanzapine-fluoxetine, and lurasidone have all demonstrated consistent efficacy in bipolar depression and are approved for this stage of the disorder.

Drug	Daily dose
Lurasidone	20–120 mg
Olanzapine-fluoxetine	6–12/25–50 mg
Quetiapine	300 mg

C – Incorrect. Consistent evidence of efficacy in bipolar depression does not exist for lamotrigine.

D – Incorrect. Consistent evidence of efficacy in bipolar depression does not exist for lamotrigine or lithium.

Reference

Bahji A, Ermacora D, Stephenson C et al. Comparative efficacy and tolerability of pharmacological treatments for the treatment of acute bipolar depression: a systematic review and network meta-analysis. *J Affect Disord* 2020;269:154–84.

QUESTION FOUR

Gina is a 24-year-old patient with no psychiatric history. She gave birth to her first child 2 weeks ago and now presents with symptoms of depression. She scores a 20 on the Edinburgh Postnatal Depression Scale (EPDS; possible depression). Which of the following courses of action should be the next step?

A. Readminister the Edinburgh Postnatal Depression Scale (EPDS) at 1 month postpartum

B. Initiate treatment with an antidepressant

C. Administer a (hypo)mania screening tool such as the Mood Disorders Questionnaire (MDQ)

Bipolar Disorder and Its Treatment

Answer to Question Four

The correct answer is C.

Choice	Peer answers
Readminister the Edinburgh Postnatal Depression Scale (EPDS) at 1 month postpartum	12%
Initiate treatment with an antidepressant	18%
Administer a (hypo)mania screening tool such as the Mood Disorders Questionnaire (MDQ)	70%

A – Incorrect. Although a follow-up administration of the EPDS may provide information on disease course, there are several great risks to untreated postpartum depression.

B – Incorrect. Although monotherapy with an antidepressant may be appropriate and effective for the treatment of postpartum depression, it is critical that patients with postpartum depression are screened for symptoms of (hypo)mania before initiating an antidepressant monotherapy that may be contraindicated.

C – Correct. Given that many patients with postpartum depression often exhibit symptoms of bipolarity or mixed features (for whom antidepressant monotherapy is not recommended), it is crucial that all patients screened as positive on the EPDS are also screened for (hypo)mania.

References

Celik SB, Bucaktepe GE, Uludag A et al. Screening mixed depression and bipolarity in the postpartum period at a primary health care center. *Compr Psychiatry* 2016;71:57–62.

Liu X, Agerbo E, Li J et al. Depression and anxiety in the postpartum period and risk of bipolar disorder: a Danish nationwide register-based cohort study. *J Clin Psychiatry* 2017;78(5):e469–76.

O'Hara MW, McCabe JE. Postpartum depression: current status and future directions. *Annu Rev Clin Psychol* 2013;9:379–407.

Sharma V, Doobay M, Baczynski C. Bipolar postpartum depression: an update and recommendations. *J Affect Disord* 2017;219:105–11.

Sharma V, Al-Farayedhi M, Doobay M et al. Should all women with postpartum depression be screened for bipolar disorder? *Med Hypotheses* 2018;118:26–8.

QUESTION FIVE

A 15-year-old girl presents with symptoms of depression. She has always been a good student and a caring and responsible sister to her two younger siblings. A few months ago, she suddenly became withdrawn and felt sad much of the time. She has had adequate trials of two different antidepressants with little improvement. Her MADRS score is currently 35, indicating severe depression. She also endorses feelings of hostility and aggression and has recently started getting into physical altercations with her peers. There is no information regarding family history as the patient is adopted. Although not definitive, this particular symptom profile may be more suggestive of:

A. Unipolar depression

B. Bipolar depression

Bipolar Disorder and Its Treatment

Answer to Question Five

The correct answer is B.

Choice	Peer answers
Unipolar depression	10%
Bipolar depression	90%

A – Incorrect. Data to date suggest that, although in no way definitive, there may be certain symptoms and course-related factors that help differentiate between unipolar and bipolar depression. This patient's presentation, which includes rapid and early onset of severe depression, hostility, aggression, and impulsivity, raises the suspicion that this may be part of a bipolar illness rather than a unipolar illness.

B – Correct. The patient's presentation includes multiple factors that may be more likely to occur with bipolar disorder rather than with unipolar depression. This is not definitive but does suggest caution when making treatment decisions. Although also not definitive, family history and input from someone close to the patient are generally more valuable than specific symptoms.

Suspect bipolar depression if:
Positive family history of bipolar disorder
Early onset of first depressive episode (<25 years)
Greater number of lifetime affective episodes
Postpartum depressive episodes
Rapid onset of depressive episodes
Greater severity of depressive episodes
Worse response to antidepressants
Antidepressant-induced hypomania
Psychotic features
Atypical depressive symptoms (e.g., leaden paralysis)
Impulsivity
Aggression
Hostility
Comorbid substance use disorder

References

Angst J, Azorin JM, Bowden CL et al. Prevalence and characteristics of undiagnosed bipolar disorders in patients with a major depressive episode: the BRIDGE study. *Arch Gen Psychiatry* 2011;68(8):791–9.

Dervic K, Garcia-Amador M, Sudol K et al. Bipolar I and II versus unipolar depression: clinical differences and impulsivity/aggression traits. *Eur Psychiatry* 2015;30(1):106–13.

Moreno C, Hasin DS, Arango C et al. Depression in bipolar disorder versus major depressive disorder: results from the National Epidemiologic Survey on Alcohol and Related Conditions. *Bipolar Disord* 2012;14:271–82.

Noto MN, de Souza Noto C, de Jesus DR et al. Recognition of bipolar disorder type I before the first manic episode: challenges and developments. *Expert Rev Neurother* 2013;13(7):795–806.

Bipolar Disorder and Its Treatment

QUESTION SIX

The "bipolar storm" refers to the concept that unstable, unregulated, and excessive neurotransmission occurs at synapses in specific brain regions, and both voltage-sensitive sodium channels and voltage-sensitive calcium channels are involved in this excessive stimulation of glutamate release. Which drugs would theoretically reduce glutamate release by blocking voltage-sensitive sodium channels?

A. Valproate and lamotrigine

B. Pregabalin and gabapentin

C. Levetiracetam and amantadine

Answer to Question Six

The correct answer is A.

Choice	Peer answers
Valproate and lamotrigine	89%
Pregabalin and gabapentin	9%
Levetiracetam and amantadine	2%

A – Correct. **Valproate** is a nonspecific voltage-sensitive sodium channel modulator and **lamotrigine** also blocks voltage-sensitive sodium channels, hypothesized to lead to reduction in glutamate release.

B – Incorrect. **Pregabalin** and **gabapentin** are alpha 2 delta ligands at voltage-sensitive calcium channels, which also leads to reduction in glutamate release.

C – Incorrect. **Levetiracetam** is a modulator of the synaptic vesicle protein SV2A, and **amantadine** is an antagonist of the N-methyl-D-aspartate (NMDA) receptor. While this combination of drugs would lead to reduced glutamate release, it would not do so via the mechanisms of action asked.

References

Sitges M, Chiu LM, Guarneros A, Nekrassov V. Effects of carbamazepine, phenytoin, lamotrigine, oxcarbazepine, topiramate, and vinpocetine on Na+ channel-mediated release of [3H]glutamate in hippocampal nerve endings. *Neuropharmacology* 2007;52(2):598–605.

Stahl SM. *Stahl's essential psychopharmacology*, fifth edition. New York, NY: Cambridge University Press; 2021. (Chapter 7)

QUESTION SEVEN

A 24-year-old man has been taking lithium for 3 years to treat his bipolar disorder. What are two primary candidates for the direct mechanisms of lithium?

A. Inhibition of glycogen synthase kinase 3β (GSK-3β) and inositol monophosphatase (IMPase)

B. Activation of GSK-3β and IMPase

C. Inhibition of GSK-3β and activation of IMPase

D. Activation of GSK-3β and inhibition of IMPase

Answer to Question Seven

The correct answer is A.

Choice	Peer answers
Inhibition of glycogen synthase kinase 3β (GSK-3β) and inositol monophosphatase (IMPase)	60%
Activation of GSK-3β and IMPase	6%
Inhibition of GSK-3β and activation of IMPase	25%
Activation of GSK-3β and inhibition of IMPase	9%

A – Correct. Lithium has been a first-line treatment for bipolar disorder for decades, yet its mechanism of action is still not certain. There is, however, substantial evidence that lithium exerts neuroprotective effects that are likely downstream from its primary mode of action. Two primary candidates for the direct mechanisms of lithium are the inhibition of GSK-3β and the inhibition of IMPase. GSK-3β is involved in the regulation of inflammation and is, in general, pro-apoptotic. Specifically, it inhibits transcription factors that would otherwise induce production of cytoprotective proteins such as brain-derived neurotrophic factor (BDNF); thus, its inhibition may be neuroprotective. IMPase indirectly leads to an increase in protein kinase C, which is overactive in mania. Thus, inhibition of IMPase by lithium could potentially reduce manic symptoms.

B – Incorrect. Lithium is thought to inhibit GSK-3β and IMPase, not activate them.

C – Incorrect. Lithium is thought to inhibit IMPase, not activate it.

D – Incorrect. Lithium is thought to inhibit GSK-3β, not activate it.

References

Malhi GS, Outhred T. Therapeutic mechanisms of lithium in bipolar disorder: recent advances and current understanding. *CNS Drugs* 2016;30(10):931–49.

Pasquali L, Busceti CL, Fulceri F, Paparelli A, Fornai F. Intracellular pathways underlying the effects of lithium. *Behav Pharmacol* 2010;21(5–6):473–92.

Won E, Kim YK. An oldie but goodie: lithium in the treatment of bipolar disorder through neuroprotective and neurotrophic mechanisms. *Int J Mol Sci* 2017;18(12):2679.

QUESTION EIGHT

Jimmy is a 20-year-old man recently diagnosed with major depressive disorder with mixed features. Approximately what percentage of patients with major depressive disorder exhibit subthreshold symptoms of (hypo)mania during a major depressive episode?

A. 6%

B. 26%

C. 46%

Answer to Question Eight

The correct answer is B.

Choice	Peer answers
6%	12%
26%	76%
46%	12%

A and C – Incorrect.

B – Correct. Approximately 26% of patients diagnosed with major depressive disorder endorse symptoms of subthreshold (hypo)mania during major depressive episodes and meet criteria for the mixed features specifier.

Reference

McIntyre RS, Soczynska JK, Cha DS et al. The prevalence and illness characteristics of DSM-5-defined "mixed feature specifier" in adults with major depressive disorder and bipolar disorder: results from the international mood disorders collaborative project. *J Affect Disord* 2015;172:259–64.

QUESTION NINE

A 24-year-old man with bipolar disorder is being initiated on lithium, with monitoring of his levels until a therapeutic serum concentration is achieved. Once the patient is stabilized, how often should his serum lithium levels be monitored (excluding one-off situations such as dose or illness change)?

A. Every 2 to 3 months

B. Every 6 to 12 months

C. Every 1 to 2 years

D. Routine monitoring is not necessary

Bipolar Disorder and Its Treatment

Answer to Question Nine

The correct answer is B.

Choice	Peer answers
Every 2 to 3 months	23%
Every 6 to 12 months	76%
Every 1 to 2 years	1%
Routine monitoring is not necessary	0%

A – Incorrect. Initially, lithium levels should be monitored every 1 to 2 weeks until the desired serum concentration is achieved, and then every 2 to 3 months for the first 6 months. However, this frequency of monitoring is not required once the patient is stabilized.

B – Correct. Once a patient is stabilized, lithium levels need only be monitored every 6 to 12 months.

C – Incorrect.

D – Incorrect.

References
Grandjean EM, Aubry JM. Lithium: updated human knowledge using an evidence-based approach. Part II: clinical pharmacology and therapeutic monitoring. *CNS Drugs* 2009;23(4):331–49.

McKnight RF, Adida M, Budge K et al. Lithium toxicity profile: a systematic review and meta-analysis. *Lancet* 2012;379:721–8.

QUESTION TEN

A 32-year-old woman with bipolar disorder has been maintained on 900 mg/day of lithium. She was doing well for a long time and had even been able to lose the weight she had initially gained with lithium. She broke up with her boyfriend 5 months ago and has been feeling depressed ever since. You augment her with 300 mg/day of quetiapine, but after several weeks she complains of weight gain and wants to change medications. Blockade of which two receptors was most likely responsible for this weight gain induced by quetiapine?

A. Muscarinic 1 and serotonin 6

B. Serotonin 2A and muscarinic 3

C. Serotonin 2C and histamine 1

D. Dopamine 2 and alpha 1 adrenergic

Answer to Question Ten

The correct answer is C.

Choice	Peer answers
Muscarinic 1 and serotonin 6	5%
Serotonin 2A and muscarinic 3	13%
Serotonin 2C and histamine 1	74%
Dopamine 2 and alpha 1 adrenergic	8%

A – Incorrect. Blockade of **muscarinic M1 receptors** can lead to constipation, blurred vision, dry mouth, and drowsiness, but not weight gain. The function of the **serotonin 6** receptors has not been identified yet.

B – Incorrect. Blockade of **serotonin 2A** receptors is considered a beneficial property of antipsychotics leading to less extrapyramidal symptoms. Blockade of **muscarinic M3** receptors has been linked to inducing cardiometabolic risk, but has not been linked to weight gain per se.

C – Correct. Blockade of **serotonin 2C** receptors and **histamine 1** receptors has been linked to weight gain.

D – Incorrect. **Dopamine 2** blockade is the main property of antipsychotics and, if continuous, this blockade can lead to motor side effects, but not to weight gain. **Alpha 1 blockade** can result in decreased blood pressure, dizziness, and drowsiness, but does not lead to weight gain.

References

Kroeze WK, Hufeisen SJ, Popadak BA et al. H1-histamine receptor affinity predicts short-term weight gain for typical and atypical antipsychotic drugs. *Neuropsychopharmacology* 2003;28(3):519–26.

Stahl SM. *Stahl's essential psychopharmacology*, fifth edition. New York, NY: Cambridge University Press; 2021. (Chapters 5, 7)

Stahl SM, Mignon L. *Stahl's illustrated antipsychotics*, second edition. New York, NY: Cambridge University Press; 2009.

QUESTION ELEVEN

Maria is a 31-year-old patient with bipolar II disorder. During major depressive episodes, this patient often experiences several symptoms of hypomania, including flight of ideas, increased risk-taking behavior, and increased talkativeness. According to data from the Stanley Foundation Bipolar Network, how many patients with bipolar disorder exhibit subsyndromal hypomanic symptoms during a major depressive episode in at least one single visit?

A. 5%

B. 25%

C. 45%

D. 65%

E. 85%

Bipolar Disorder and Its Treatment

Answer to Question Eleven

The correct answer is D.

Choice	Peer answers
5%	1%
25%	44%
45%	22%
65%	32%
85%	1%

A, B, C, and E – Incorrect.

D – Correct. According to data published by the Stanley Foundation Bipolar Network, as many as 65% of patients with bipolar disorder exhibit symptoms of subsyndromal hypomania during depressive episodes at a single visit.

Reference

Miller S, Suppes T, Mintz J et al. Mixed depression in bipolar disorder: prevalence rate and clinical correlates during naturalistic follow-up in the Stanley Bipolar Network. *Am J Psychiatry* 2016;173(10):1015–23.

QUESTION TWELVE

Thomas, a 28-year-old patient with major depressive disorder with mixed features, complains of significant irritability and agitation that are affecting his family and work. Which psychotropic treatment(s) can be considered as ALTERNATIVE maintenance treatments to antidepressants?

A. An atypical antipsychotic such as quetiapine

B. A mood stabilizer such as lamotrigine

C. A benzodiazepine such as lorazepam

D. A and B only

E. B and C only

Answer to Question Twelve

The correct answer is D.

Choice	Peer answers
An atypical antipsychotic such as quetiapine	9%
A mood stabilizer such as lamotrigine	4%
A benzodiazepine such as lorazepam	1%
A and B only	86%
B and C only	1%

A – Partially correct. Atypical antipsychotics with mood-stabilizing properties (such as quetiapine) are recommended as first-line treatments in patients with major depressive disorder with mixed features.

B – Partially correct. Mood stabilizers (such as lamotrigine) are recommended as first- or second-line treatments in patients with major depressive disorder with mixed features.

C and E – Incorrect. Although benzodiazepines (such as lorazepam) may be useful for reducing acute mania, there are no data supporting the use of benzodiazepines in the maintenance treatment of major depressive disorder with mixed features. Additionally, the extended use of benzodiazepines is not recommended due to high risk for dependence, tolerance, and withdrawal.

D – Correct. Both atypical antipsychotics with mood-stabilizing properties and mood stabilizers have shown some efficacy in the treatment of major depressive episodes with mixed features and are therefore recommended as first- or second-line treatments.

References

McIntyre RS, Lee Y, Mansur RB. A pragmatic approach to the diagnosis and treatment of mixed features in adults with mood disorders. *CNS Spectr* 2016;21:28–32.

Stahl SM. *Essential psychopharmacology, the prescriber's guide*, seventh edition. New York, NY: Cambridge University Press; 2020.

Stahl SM, Morrissette DA, Faedda G et al. Guidelines for the recognition and treatment of mixed depression. *CNS Spectr* 2017;22(2):203–19.

QUESTION THIRTEEN

A 21-year-old patient with major depressive disorder presents with several symptoms that may indicate the presence of mixed features. Which of the following symptoms is included in the DSM-5 mixed features specifier diagnostic criteria?

A. Irritability

B. Increased goal-directed activity

C. Distractibility

D. Agitation

Bipolar Disorder and Its Treatment

Answer to Question Thirteen

The correct answer is B.

Choice	Peer answers
Irritability	35%
Increased goal-directed activity	47%
Distractibility	3%
Agitation	15%

B – Correct. Although increased goal-directed activity is NOT one of the most common symptoms exhibited by patients experiencing a major depressive episode with mixed features, it is included in the DSM-5 mixed features specifier diagnostic criteria.

A, C, and D – Incorrect. Although irritability, distractibility, and psychomotor agitation are among the most common symptoms of depression with mixed features, they are excluded from the DSM-5 mixed features criteria due to the overlap of these symptoms with other disorders (e.g., anxiety disorders) and between mania and depression.

References

Koukopoulos A, Sani G. DSM-5 criteria for depression with mixed features: a farewell to mixed depression. *Acta Psychiatr Scand* 2014;129:4–16.

Mahli GS, Laampe L, Coulston CM et al. Mixed state discrimination: a DSM problem that won't go away? *J Affect Disord* 2014;158:8–10.

Takeshima M, Oka T. DSM-5-defined "mixed features" and Benazzi's mixed depression: which is practically useful to discriminate bipolar disorder from unipolar depression in patients with depression? *Psychiatry Clin Neurosci* 2015;69(2):109–16.

Bipolar Disorder and Its Treatment

QUESTION FOURTEEN

A patient with bipolar depression has been treated for 6 months with lamotrigine plus an atypical antipsychotic with partial response. The decision is made to stop the atypical antipsychotic; however, during down-titration, the patient develops withdrawal dyskinesias. No treatment for the dyskinesias is initiated, and after 2 weeks they still remain. Which of the following is true?

A. If the withdrawal dyskinesias still remain after 2 weeks, they are likely to be permanent

B. The patient's withdrawal dyskinesias may take several weeks to months to resolve

Bipolar Disorder and Its Treatment

Answer to Question Fourteen

The correct answer is B.

Choice	Peer answers
If the withdrawal dyskinesias still remain after 2 weeks, they are likely to be permanent	11%
The patient's withdrawal dyskinesias may take several weeks to months to resolve	89%

A – Incorrect. Withdrawal dyskinesias are often reversible with time and usually resolve within a few weeks; however, they can take several months to resolve, depending on their seriousness. Thus, although the patient's withdrawal dyskinesias still remain after 2 weeks, this does not indicate that they are likely to be permanent.

B – Correct. It may take several weeks to months for the patient's withdrawal dyskinesias to resolve.

References
Aia PG, Reveulta GJ, Cloud LJ, Factor SA. Tardive dyskinesia. *Curr Treat Options Neurol* 2011;13(3):231–41.

Moseley CN, Simpson-Khanna HA, Catalano G, Catalano MC. Covert dyskinesia associated with aripiprazole: a case report and review of the literature. *Clin Neuropharmacol* 2013;36(4):128–30.

Umbrich P, Soares KV. Benzodiazepines for neuroleptic-induced tardive dyskinesia. *Cochrane Database Syst Rev* 2003;(2):CD000205.

QUESTION FIFTEEN

A 38-year-old patient with bipolar disorder has been taking valproate with only partial control of depressive symptoms, and her clinician elects to add lamotrigine. Compared to lamotrigine monotherapy, what adjustment should be made to the lamotrigine titration schedule in the presence of valproate?

A. Slower titration schedule, half the target dose

B. Slower titration schedule, same target dose

C. Same titration schedule, half the target dose

D. Same titration schedule, same dose

Answer to Question Fifteen

The correct answer is A.

Choice	Peer answers
Slower titration schedule, half the target dose	72%
Slower titration schedule, same target dose	9%
Same titration schedule, half the target dose	17%
Same titration schedule, same dose	2%

A – Correct. Valproate increases the plasma levels of lamotrigine, so when adding lamotrigine to valproate, the target dose is lower and titration is slower (in comparison to initiating lamotrigine monotherapy):

- For the first 2 weeks: 25 mg every other day
- Week 3: increase to 25 mg/day
- Week 5: increase to 50 mg/day
- Week 6: increase to 100 mg/day

B, C, and D – Incorrect.

Reference

Stahl SM. *Essential psychopharmacology, the prescriber's guide*, seventh edition. New York, NY: Cambridge University Press; 2020.

QUESTION SIXTEEN

A 28-year-old obese woman presents with a depressive episode. She has previously been hospitalized and treated for a manic episode but is not currently taking any medication. Of the following, the agent with the lowest risk of cardiometabolic side effects is:

A. Lithium

B. Lumateperone

C. Olanzapine

D. Valproate

Answer to Question Sixteen

The correct answer is B.

Choice	Peer answers
Lithium	24%
Lumateperone	58%
Olanzapine	6%
Valproate	12%

A, C, and D – Incorrect. Both lithium and valproate are associated with a relatively high risk of significant weight gain. Among the atypical antipsychotics, olanzapine carries with it one of the highest risks for cardiometabolic side effects, including weight gain.

B – Correct. Lumateperone has been shown to be neutral for weight gain in long-term studies and in early clinical practice, and has a favorable metabolic profile that is similar to placebo for changes in triglycerides, fasting glucose, and cholesterol.

References

Stahl SM. *Stahl's essential psychopharmacology, the prescriber's guide*, seventh edition. New York, NY: Cambridge University Press; 2020.

Yalin N, Young AH. Pharmacological treatment of bipolar depression: what are the current and emerging options? *Neuropsychiatr Dis Treat* 2020;9(16):1459–72.

QUESTION SEVENTEEN

Patricia is a 31-year-old patient with bipolar I disorder who frequently exhibits impulsive symptoms of mania, including risk taking and pressured speech, during her manic episodes. Compared to a healthy brain, neuroimaging of this patient's brain during a no-go task (designed to test response inhibition) would likely show:

A. Increased activity in the orbitofrontal cortex

B. Decreased activity in the orbitofrontal cortex

C. Increased activity in the dorsolateral prefrontal cortex

Answer to Question Seventeen

The correct answer is B.

Choice	Peer answers
Increased activity in the orbitofrontal cortex	23%
Decreased activity in the orbitofrontal cortex	53%
Increased activity in the dorsolateral prefrontal cortex	24%

A – Incorrect. Compared to healthy controls, neuroimaging studies indicate that the orbitofrontal cortex is hypoactive while performing a no-go task in patients with mania.

B – Correct. Neuroimaging of the orbitofrontal cortex of manic patients during a no-go task (a task that required the patient to suppress a response) shows that they fail to appropriately activate this brain region. This neuroimaging anomaly suggests that patients with bipolar disorder have problems with impulsivity associated with mania and with the orbitofrontal cortex.

C – Incorrect. Neuroimaging studies indicate that resting activity in the dorsolateral prefrontal cortex of depressed patients is decreased compared to healthy controls. However, there are no data indicating an elevation in activity in the dorsolateral prefrontal cortex during a no-go task in patients with mania.

References
Elliot R, Ogilvie A, Rubinsztein JS et al. Abnormal ventral frontal response during performance of an affective go/no go task in patients with mania. *Biol Psychiatry* 2004;155(12):1163–70.

Price JL, Drevets WC. Neurocircuitry of mood disorders. *Neuropsychopharmacology* 2010;35(1):192–216.

Stahl SM. *Stahl's essential psychopharmacology*, fifth edition. New York, NY: Cambridge University Press; 2021. (Chapter 6)

QUESTION EIGHTEEN

Katherine is a 24-year-old patient who presents with symptoms of depression (including sadness, feelings of worthlessness, and suicidal ideation) occurring every day for the past month. Clinical interview with Katherine reveals that she has a maternal aunt with bipolar disorder I. Further assessment reveals that this patient also feels distracted and as though her thoughts are racing. Upon speaking with the patient's mother, it is discovered that Katherine has been, at times, more talkative than usual and irritable with her friends and family. Which class of medication would *not* be recommended as monotherapy for this patient?

A. A mood stabilizer

B. An antipsychotic

C. An antidepressant

D. All of the above would be recommended as monotherapy

Answer to Question Eighteen

The correct answer is C.

Choice	Peer answers
A mood stabilizer	1%
An antipsychotic	2%
An antidepressant	95%
All of the above would be recommended as monotherapy	2%

A – Incorrect. Expert consensus and published guidelines recommend that patients who exhibit mixed features during a major depressive episode and positive family history of bipolar disorder be treated with a mood stabilizer as a first- or second-line treatment strategy.

B – Incorrect. Expert consensus and published guidelines recommend that patients who exhibit mixed features during a major depressive episode and positive family history of bipolar disorder be treated with an atypical antipsychotic that has evidence of mood-stabilizing properties (e.g., lurasidone, quetiapine) as a first- or second-line treatment strategy.

C – Correct. Expert consensus and published guidelines recommend that antidepressant monotherapy *not* be used (and is contraindicated) in patients with depression who exhibit mixed features and a positive family history of bipolar disorder.

D – Incorrect.

References
Pompili M, **Vazquez GH**, **Forte A** et al. Pharmacologic treatment of mixed states. *Psychiatr Clin North Am* 2020;43(1):167–86.

Stahl SM, **Morrissette DA**. Does a "whiff" of mania in a major depressive episode shift treatment from a classical antidepressant to an atypical/second-generation antipsychotic? *Bipolar Disord* 2017;19(7):595–6.

Stahl SM, **Morrissette DA**, **Faedda G** et al. Guidelines for the recognition and management of mixed depression. *CNS Spectr* 2017;22(2):203–19.

QUESTION NINETEEN

Stacey is a 25-year-old patient with bipolar depression, who tends to endorse some manic symptoms during depressive episodes. Of the following symptoms, which is the most common subsyndromal mania symptom in patients during a major depressive episode with mixed features?

A. Decreased need for sleep

B. Inflated self-esteem

C. Psychomotor agitation

D. Elevated mood

E. High-risk behavior

Answer to Question Nineteen

The correct answer is C.

Choice	Peer answers
Decreased need for sleep	25%
Inflated self-esteem	2%
Psychomotor agitation	58%
Elevated mood	4%
High-risk behavior	12%

A, B, D, and E – Incorrect. Decreased need for sleep, inflated self-esteem, elevated mood, and high-risk behavior are among the manic symptoms most rarely seen in patients with mixed features during a major depressive episode.

C – Correct. During a major depressive episode with mixed features (concomitant subthreshold levels of mania or hypomania), the most common manic/hypomanic symptom exhibited is psychomotor agitation.

References

Koukopoulos A, Sani G. DSM-5 criteria for depression with mixed features: a farewell to mixed depression. *Acta Psychiatr Scand* 2014;129:4–16.

Mahli GS, Laampe L, Coulston CM et al. Mixed state discrimination: a DSM problem that won't go away? *J Affect Disord* 2014;158:8–10.

Takeshima M, Oka T. DSM-5-defined "mixed features" and Benazzi's mixed depression: which is practically useful to discriminate bipolar disorder from unipolar depression in patients with depression? *Psychiatry Clin Neurosci* 2015;69(2):109–16.

QUESTION TWENTY

Hilary is a 22-year-old patient with bipolar disorder and comorbid attention deficit hyperactivity disorder (ADHD). Approximately what percentage of patients with bipolar disorder have comorbid ADHD?

A. 1–2%

B. 20–25%

C. 40–50%

Answer to Question Twenty

The correct answer is B.

Choice	Peer answers
1–2%	3%
20–25%	84%
40–50%	13%

A and C – Incorrect.

B – Correct. Approximately 20–25% of patients with bipolar disorder have comorbid ADHD.

References

Kessler RC, Adler L, Barkley R et al. The prevalence and correlates of adult ADHD in the United States: results from the National Comorbidity Survey Replication. *Am J Psychiatry* 2006;163(4):716–23.

Perroud N, Cordera P, Zimmermann J et al. Comorbidity between attention deficit hyperactivity disorder (ADHD) and bipolar disorder in a specialized mood disorders outpatient clinic. *J Affect Disord* 2014;168:161–6.

Pinna M, Visioli C, Rago CM et al. Attention deficit-hyperactivity disorder in adult bipolar disorder patients. *J Affect Disord* 2019;243:391–6.

CHAPTER PEER COMPARISON

For the Bipolar Disorder section, the correct answer was selected 75% of the time.

5 CHRONIC NEUROPATHIC PAIN AND ITS TREATMENT

QUESTION ONE

A 34-year-old woman with fibromyalgia, generalized anxiety disorder, and depression is currently taking several psychotropic medications, including alprazolam, duloxetine, hydrocodone/acetaminophen, and pregabalin. She continues to have residual pain, anxiety, and mood symptoms. Her clinician is considering simplifying her medication regimen and plans to discontinue the medication with the least evidence of efficacy for her disorders. Which of the following should be discontinued?

A. Alprazolam

B. Duloxetine

C. Hydrocodone/acetaminophen

D. Pregabalin

Answer to Question One

The correct answer is C.

Choice	Peer answers
Alprazolam	27%
Duloxetine	2%
Hydrocodone/acetaminophen	69%
Pregabalin	2%

A – Incorrect. Alprazolam is an effective treatment for generalized anxiety disorder.

B – Incorrect. Duloxetine is an effective treatment for both depression and for fibromyalgia.

C – Correct. Hydrocodone/acetaminophen does not have evidence of efficacy for the treatment of fibromyalgia, nor is it an appropriate treatment for her other illnesses.

D – Incorrect. Pregabalin is an effective treatment for fibromyalgia and also has evidence of efficacy in anxiety.

References

Ballantyne JC, Shin NS. Efficacy of opioids for chronic pain: a review of the evidence. *Clin J Pain* 2008;24:469–78.

Clauw DJ. Fibromyalgia: an overview. *Am J Med* 2009;122(12 Suppl): S3–13.

Chronic Neuropathic Pain and Its Treatment

QUESTION TWO

A 35-year-old woman complains of widespread pain so debilitating that she has been unable to work for the last several weeks, though she did not experience any significant injury that seems to account for the pain. Specifically, she states that even the mild pressure of being touched causes such significant pain that she cringes when her 2-year-old daughter tries to hug her. This type of pain is called:

A. Acute pain

B. Allodynia

C. Hyperalgesia

Answer to Question Two

The correct answer is B.

Choice	Peer answers
Acute pain	1%
Allodynia	55%
Hyperalgesia	44%

A – Incorrect. Acute pain refers to pain that resolves after a short duration and that is usually directly related to tissue damage. In this case the patient has had significant pain for several weeks despite the lack of any apparent injury; thus, this does not appear to be acute pain.

B – Correct. Allodynia is a painful response to a stimulus that does not normally provoke pain, such as pain in response to light touch. This is consistent with what the patient describes.

C – Incorrect. Hyperalgesia is an exaggerated pain response to something that is normally painful (for example, extreme pain in response to a pin prick). Mild pressure from being hugged by one's child would not normally elicit pain, and thus this particular complaint does not represent hyperalgesia.

References

Kumar A, Kaur H, Singh A. Neuropathic pain models caused by damage to central or peripheral nervous system. *Pharmacol Rep* 2018;70(2):206–16.

Stahl SM. *Stahl's essential psychopharmacology*, fifth edition. New York, NY: Cambridge University Press; 2021. (Chapter 9)

QUESTION THREE

A young man arrives at the emergency room in great pain after receiving a chemical burn during an accident at work. Which primary afferent neurons would have responded to the chemical stimulus to produce nociceptive neuronal activity?

A. A-beta fiber neurons

B. A-delta fiber neurons

C. C fiber neurons

Answer to Question Three

The correct answer is C.

Choice	Peer answers
A-beta fiber neurons	16%
A-delta fiber neurons	28%
C fiber neurons	56%

A – Incorrect. A-beta fibers respond to non-noxious small movements such as light touch, hair movement, and vibrations, and do not respond to noxious stimuli.

B – Incorrect. A-delta fibers fall somewhere in between A-beta fibers and C fiber neurons, sensing noxious mechanical stimuli and sub-noxious thermal stimuli.

C – Correct. C fiber peripheral terminals are bare nerve endings that are only activated by noxious mechanical, thermal, or chemical stimuli. Thus, C fiber neurons are the primary afferent neurons responsible for nociceptive conduction following this patient's injury.

References

Kumar A, Kaur H, Singh A. Neuropathic pain models caused by damage to central or peripheral nervous system. *Pharmacol Rep* 2018;70(2):206–16.

Stahl SM. *Stahl's essential psychopharmacology*, fifth edition. New York, NY: Cambridge University Press; 2021. (Chapter 9)

QUESTION FOUR

Pain experienced by patients that is not associated with signs of neuropathy, but is characterized by hypersensitivity in apparently normal tissues is called:

A. Inflammatory

B. Neuropathic

C. Nociplastic

D. Nociceptive

Answer to Question Four

The correct answer is C.

Choice	Peer answers
Inflammatory	6%
Neuropathic	15%
Nociplastic	35%
Nociceptive	43%

A and D – Incorrect. Inflammatory, or nociceptive, pain is pain in response to an injury or stimulus. Examples of this type of pain include injuries, bruises, burns, arthritis, and sprains.

B – Incorrect. Neuropathic pain develops when the nervous system is damaged due to a lesion or disease. Examples of this type of pain include postherpetic neuralgia, trigeminal neuralgia, neuropathic low back pain.

C – Correct. In 2018, the International Association for the Study of Pain (IASP) proposed the term "nociplastic" for pain that results from altered nociception despite no clear evidence of actual or threatened tissue damage or evidence of a lesion or disease. Nociplastic pain is chronic, and types of nociplastic pain include fibromyalgia, irritable bowel syndrome, complex regional pain syndrome, and nonspecific chronic low back pain.

References

Aydede M, Shriver A. Recently introduced definition of "nociplastic pain" by the International Association for the Study of Pain needs better formulation. *Pain* 2018;159:1176–7.

Kosek E, Cohen M, Baron R et al. Do we need a third mechanistic descriptor for chronic pain states? *Pain* 2016;157:1382–6.

Kumar A, Kaur H, Singh A. Neuropathic pain models caused by damage to central or peripheral nervous system. *Pharmacol Rep* 2018;70(2):206–16.

QUESTION FIVE

A 29-year-old woman has just been diagnosed with major depressive disorder and is being prescribed a selective serotonin reuptake inhibitor (SSRI). In addition to depressed mood, lack of interest in her work or friends, and difficulty sleeping, she has been experiencing aches and pains in her arms, shoulders, and torso. She asks if the SSRI is likely to alleviate her painful physical symptoms as well as her emotional ones. Which of the following statements is true?

A. SSRIs may have inconsistent effects on pain because serotonin can both inhibit and facilitate ascending nociceptive signals

B. SSRIs may worsen pain because serotonin can facilitate but not inhibit ascending nociceptive signals

C. SSRIs generally alleviate pain because serotonin can inhibit but not facilitate ascending nociceptive signals

D. SSRIs generally have no effect on pain because serotonin neither facilitates nor inhibits nociceptive signals

Chronic Neuropathic Pain and Its Treatment

Answer to Question Five

The correct answer is A.

Choice	Peer answers
SSRIs may have inconsistent effects on pain because serotonin can both inhibit and facilitate ascending nociceptive signals	60%
SSRIs may worsen pain because serotonin can facilitate but not inhibit ascending nociceptive signals	1%
SSRIs generally alleviate pain because serotonin can inhibit but not facilitate ascending nociceptive signals	16%
SSRIs generally have no effect on pain because serotonin neither facilitates nor inhibits nociceptive signals	24%

Two important descending pathways that inhibit ascending nociceptive signals are the noradrenergic and the serotonergic pathways. Thus, enhancement of neurotransmission in either of these pathways could contribute to alleviation of chronic pain.

However, serotonin is also a major neurotransmitter in descending facilitation pathways to the spinal cord. The combination of both inhibitory and facilitatory actions of serotonin may explain why SSRIs seem to have inconsistent effects on painful somatic symptoms.

A – Correct. SSRIs may have inconsistent effects on pain because serotonin can both inhibit and facilitate ascending nociceptive signals.

B, C, and D – Incorrect.

References
Belinskaia DA, Belinskaia MA, Barygin OI, Vanchakova NP, Shestakova NN. Psychotropic drugs for the management of chronic pain and itch. *Pharmaceuticals (Basel)* 2019;12(2):99.

Stahl SM. *Stahl's essential psychopharmacology*, fifth edition. New York, NY: Cambridge University Press; 2021. (Chapter 9)

QUESTION SIX

A 22-year-old woman with pain throughout her body, extreme fatigue, and poor sleep is diagnosed with fibromyalgia. Her care provider considers prescribing pregabalin, which may alleviate pain by:

A. Binding to the closed conformation of voltage-sensitive sodium channels

B. Binding to the open conformation of voltage-sensitive sodium channels

C. Binding to the closed conformation of voltage-sensitive calcium channels

D. Binding to the open conformation of voltage-sensitive calcium channels

Chronic Neuropathic Pain and Its Treatment

Answer to Question Six

The correct answer is D.

Choice	Peer answers
Binding to the closed conformation of voltage-sensitive sodium channels	10%
Binding to the open conformation of voltage-sensitive sodium channels	21%
Binding to the closed conformation of voltage-sensitive calcium channels	17%
Binding to the open conformation of voltage-sensitive calcium channels	52%

A and B – Incorrect. Both voltage-sensitive sodium channels and voltage-sensitive calcium channels (VSCCs) are involved in transmission of pain; however, pregabalin does not bind to voltage-sensitive sodium channels in any conformation.

C – Incorrect. This molecular action predicts more affinity for VSCCs that are actively conducting neuronal impulses within the pain pathway, and thus a selective action on those VSCCs causing neuropathic pain, ignoring other VSCCs that are closed, and thus not interfering with normal neurotransmission in central neurons uninvolved in mediating the pathological pain state.

D – Correct. Pregabalin does, however, bind to the alpha 2 delta subunit of VSCCs. In fact, pregabalin binds preferentially to the open conformation of these channels and thus may be particularly effective in blocking channels that are the most active, with a "use-dependent" form of inhibition.

References
Dooley DJ, Taylor CP, Donevan S, Feltner D. Ca^{2+} channel alpha 2 delta ligands: novel modulators of neurotransmission. *Trends Pharmacol Sci* 2007;28:75–82.

Jensen TS. Anticonvulsants in neuropathic pain: rationale and clinical evidence. *Eur J Pain* 2002;6(Suppl A):61–8.

Stahl SM. *Stahl's essential psychopharmacology*, fifth edition. New York, NY: Cambridge University Press; 2021. (Chapter 9)

QUESTION SEVEN

A 34-year-old man with juvenile-onset diabetes has begun experiencing throbbing pain, particularly at night. In addition, he states that his body generally feels sensitive all over, so that even the brush of his clothes against his skin can be uncomfortable. These symptoms, indicative of diabetic peripheral neuropathy, may be caused by:

A. Inflammation or damage in the periphery without disturbance in central pain processing

B. Central disturbance in pain processing without damage in the periphery

C. Inflammation or damage in the periphery combined with central disturbance in pain processing

Answer to Question Seven

The correct answer is C.

Choice	Peer answers
Inflammation or damage in the periphery without disturbance in central pain processing	20%
Central disturbance in pain processing without damage in the periphery	5%
Inflammation or damage in the periphery combined with central disturbance in pain processing	76%

A and B – Incorrect.

C – Correct. Chronic pain syndromes may be peripheral, central, or both peripheral and central ("mixed") in origin. Over time, diabetes can cause inflammation that damages peripheral nerves and thus leads to painful physical symptoms. In addition, that damage may cause repetitive activation of nociception, and such ongoing neuronal activity may induce central plasticity within the pain pathway, with progressive and potentially irreversible molecular changes in pain processing pathways eventually leading to progressive and potentially irreversible pain symptoms. Thus, diabetic peripheral neuropathy is a syndrome in which definite peripheral injury is combined with central sensitization.

References

Fernandes V, Sharma D, Vaidya S et al. Cellular and molecular mechanisms driving neuropathic pain: recent advancements and challenges. *Expert Opin Ther Targets* 2018;22(2):131–42.

Kumar A, Kaur H, Singh A. Neuropathic pain models caused by damage to central or peripheral nervous system. *Pharmacol Rep* 2018;70(2):206–16.

Stahl SM. *Stahl's essential psychopharmacology*, fifth edition. New York, NY: Cambridge University Press; 2021. (Chapter 9)

QUESTION EIGHT

A 34-year-old man presents with chronic back pain and a major depressive episode. Which of the following are documented to treat both chronic central pain and depression without significant side effects?

A. Amitriptyline

B. Duloxetine

C. Gabapentin

D. Sertraline

Answer to Question Eight

The correct answer is B.

Choice	Peer answers
Amitriptyline	3%
Duloxetine	91%
Gabapentin	5%
Sertraline	1%

A – Incorrect. Although effective for depression and chronic pain, tricyclic antidepressants such as amitriptyline have several unwanted mechanisms. Histamine 1 receptor blockade causes sedation and may lead to weight gain. Muscarinic M1 receptor blockade causes dry mouth, blurred vision, urinary retention, and constipation; and muscarinic M3 receptor blockade can interfere with insulin action. Alpha 1 adrenergic receptor blockade causes orthostatic hypotension and dizziness.

B – Correct. Duloxetine, a serotonin norepinephrine reuptake inhibitor (SNRI), may be the antidepressant that is best documented to have efficacy in pain conditions. Duloxetine targets both descending noradrenergic and serotonergic projections and the patient may benefit from an antidepressant with dual mechanisms, which may help alleviate his chronic pain.

C – Incorrect. Gabapentin, an alpha 2 delta ligand, is not documented to show efficacy in the treatment of depression.

D – Incorrect. Sertraline, a selective serotonin reuptake inhibitor (SSRI), is not documented to treat chronic central pain. It is also possible that the patient may benefit instead from an antidepressant treatment with dual mechanisms, particularly one with noradrenergic properties, which may help alleviate his chronic pain.

References

Stahl SM. *Stahl's essential psychopharmacology: the prescriber's guide*, seventh edition. New York, NY: Cambridge University Press; 2020.

Stahl SM. *Stahl's essential psychopharmacology*, fifth edition. New York, NY: Cambridge University Press; 2021. (Chapter 9)

QUESTION NINE

A 36-year-old woman has just been diagnosed with fibromyalgia. In addition to her painful physical symptoms, she is experiencing problems with memory and significant difficulty concentrating at work. Which of the following may be most likely to alleviate both her physical pain and her cognitive symptoms?

A. Bupropion

B. Cyclobenzaprine

C. Milnacipran

D. Pregabalin

Chronic Neuropathic Pain and Its Treatment

Answer to Question Nine

The correct answer is C.

Choice	Peer answers
Bupropion	21%
Cyclobenzaprine	2%
Milnacipran	55%
Pregabalin	21%

Documented mechanisms for alleviating central neuropathic pain include enhancement of serotonergic and noradrenergic neurotransmission in descending spinal pathways as well as reduction of calcium influx in pain pathways. Cognitive dysfunction may be alleviated by increasing dopaminergic (and possibly noradrenergic) neurotransmission in the dorsolateral prefrontal cortex.

A – Incorrect. Bupropion is a norepinephrine and dopamine reuptake inhibitor (NDRI) and may reduce cognitive symptoms associated with fibromyalgia when used as adjunct but is not documented to reduce pain.

B – Incorrect. Cyclobenzaprine is a muscle relaxant and may be used for fibromyalgia but is not generally a first-line choice and does not have efficacy for cognitive symptoms.

C – Correct. Milnacipran is a serotonin norepinephrine reuptake inhibitor (SNRI) with documented efficacy for treating neuropathic pain. In addition, it can also improve cognitive symptoms through its potent norepinephrine reuptake binding property.

D – Incorrect. Pregabalin binds to the alpha 2 delta subunit of voltage-sensitive calcium channels to reduce calcium influx. It has documented efficacy for treating neuropathic pain but is not documented to reduce cognitive symptoms.

References

Stahl SM. *Case studies: Stahl's essential psychopharmacology*. New York, NY: Cambridge University Press; 2011.

Stahl SM. *Stahl's essential psychopharmacology*, fifth edition. New York, NY: Cambridge University Press; 2021. (Chapter 9)

QUESTION TEN

A 44-year-old male patient with chronic hepatitis is seeking treatment for chronic neuropathic pain. Which of the following would you most likely avoid prescribing for this patient?

A. Duloxetine

B. Gabapentin

C. Pregabalin

Chronic Neuropathic Pain and Its Treatment

Answer to Question Ten

The correct answer is A.

Choice	Peer answers
Duloxetine	68%
Gabapentin	18%
Pregabalin	14%

All of these medications can be effective for chronic neuropathic pain; what distinguishes them here is their effects in hepatic impairment.

A – Correct. Duloxetine increases the risk of elevation of serum transaminase levels and is not recommended for use in individuals with hepatic insufficiency; thus, it would not be recommended in this case.

B and C – Incorrect. Gabapentin and pregabalin are not metabolized by the liver, nor do they appear to have effects on liver functioning; thus, they are considered safe in hepatic impairment and do not generally require dose adjustment.

References

Atkinson JH, Slater MA, Capparelli EV et al. Efficacy of noradrenergic and serotonergic antidepressants in chronic back pain: a preliminary concentration-controlled trial. *J Clin Psychopharmacol* 2007;27:135–42.

Scholz BA, Hammonds CL, Boomershine CS. Duloxetine for the management of fibromyalgia syndrome. *J Pain Res* 2009;2:99–108.

Stahl SM. *Stahl's essential psychopharmacology: the prescriber's guide*, seventh edition. New York, NY: Cambridge University Press; 2020.

QUESTION ELEVEN

Sarah is a 42-year-old patient with long-standing abdominal pain attributed to Crohn's disease, as well as low back pain with associated insomnia and depression. She is currently on 30 mg oral methadone three times a day, 60 mg duloxetine once a day, and 10 mg desipramine at bedtime. Which of the following opioid analgesic drugs may have the lowest risk for Sarah developing serotonin syndrome?

A. Meperidine

B. Methadone

C. Morphine

D. Tramadol

Chronic Neuropathic Pain and Its Treatment

Answer to Question Eleven

The correct answer is C.

Choice	Peer answers
Meperidine	14%
Methadone	19%
Morphine	50%
Tramadol	18%

In the presence of other serotonergic agents, opioids may significantly affect serotonin kinetics, causing increased intrasynaptic serotonin levels, which can lead to the development of serotonin syndrome. In March 2016, the US Food and Drug Administration (FDA) issued a warning about the potential interaction between opioids and antidepressants and the development of serotonin syndrome.

A – Incorrect. Meperidine is a potent inhibitor of serotonin reuptake and toxic reactions have been known to occur when meperidine is given to patients on monoamine oxidase inhibitor (MAOI) or tricyclic antidepressant therapy.

B – Incorrect. Methadone has an inhibitory effect on serotonin transporters. Serotonin syndrome has been reported in a few cases when methadone therapy is co-administered with a selective serotonin reuptake inhibitor (SSRI).

C – Correct. Certain synthetic opioids such as tramadol, methadone, meperidine, fentanyl, and dextromethorphan are weak serotonin reuptake inhibitors and can cause toxicity, but opioids with a structure similar to morphine are not reuptake inhibitors and may be less likely to cause serotonin syndrome (or serotonin toxicity).

D – Incorrect. Tramadol is a racemic mixture of R and S enantiomers. The R enantiomer is a mu-opioid receptor agonist, while the S enantiomer inhibits reuptake of norepinephrine and releases serotonin, which results in an excess of intrasynaptic serotonin when combined with other serotonergic drugs.

The list of clinical features for serotonin syndrome, ranging from mild to severe, is often viewed as a triad of changes in neuromuscular hyperactivity (clonus, hyperreflexia, myoclonus, and rigidity in advanced stages of toxicity), autonomic nervous system hyperactivity (hyperthermia, tachycardia, diaphoresis, and mydriasis), and changes in mental status (agitation, excitement, restlessness, and confusion in advanced stages).

References

Baldo BA, Rose MA. The anaesthetist, opioid analgesic drugs, and serotonin toxicity: a mechanistic and clinical review. *Br J Anaesth* 2020;124(1):44–62.

Francescangeli J, Karamchandani K, Powell M, Bonavia A. The serotonin syndrome: from molecular mechanisms to clinical practice. *Int J Mol Sci* 2019;20(9):2288.

US Food and Drug Administration. FDA Drug Safety Communication: FDA warns about several safety issues with opioid pain medicines; requires label changes. March 22, 2016.

Chronic Neuropathic Pain and Its Treatment

QUESTION TWELVE

Which of the following statements about the use of antidepressants for pain management is correct?

A. They relieve pain primarily in patients with depression

B. They relieve pain at higher doses than those used for an anti-depressant effect

C. They may relieve pain by blocking receptors for serotonin and norepinephrine in the central nervous system (CNS)

D. They may relieve pain by blocking the reuptake of serotonin and norepinephrine in the CNS

Chronic Neuropathic Pain and Its Treatment

Answer to Question Twelve

The correct answer is D.

Choice	Peer answers
They relieve pain primarily in patients with depression	4%
They relieve pain at higher doses than those used for an antidepressant effect	8%
They may relieve pain by blocking receptors for serotonin and norepinephrine in the central nervous system (CNS)	9%
They may relieve pain by blocking the reuptake of serotonin and norepinephrine in the CNS	80%

A – Incorrect. Antidepressants have not been shown to provide more relief for patients with depression compared to others.

B – Incorrect. The doses for antidepressants that are effective for pain are generally lower than the doses used for depression.

C – Incorrect.

D – Correct. The mechanism of action of the antidepressants is that they inhibit the reuptake of the biogenic amines, mostly norepinephrine as well as serotonin, which hypothetically increases the presence of these neurotransmitters to increase nociceptive inhibition.

References

Atkinson JH, Slater MA, Capparelli EV et al. Efficacy of noradrenergic and serotonergic antidepressants in chronic back pain: a preliminary concentration-controlled trial. *J Clin Psychopharmacol* 2007;27:35–142.

Belinskaia DA, Belinskaia MA, Barygin OI, Vanchakova NP, Shestakova NN. Psychotropic drugs for the management of chronic pain and itch. *Pharmaceuticals (Basel)* 2019;12(2):99.

Stahl SM. *Stahl's essential psychopharmacology*, fifth edition. New York, NY: Cambridge University Press; 2021. (Chapter 9)

CHAPTER PEER COMPARISON

For the Chronic Neuropathic Pain section, the correct answer was selected 62% of the time.

6 DEMENTIA AND ITS TREATMENT

QUESTION ONE

Harold, a 74-year-old patient, is brought to your office by his daughter, who reports that her father has been exhibiting several concerning symptoms over the past year. Comprehensive questioning reveals that his symptoms are: trouble remembering familiar things, such as telephone numbers commonly dialed; not recognizing some close family members who visit often; and difficulty performing writing tasks. The patient's motor function appears to be unaffected. Although not definitive, these symptoms are most likely indicative of which type of dementia?

A. Alzheimer's disease

B. Frontotemporal dementia

C. Huntington's disease

Answer to Question One

The correct answer is A.

Choice	Peer answers
Alzheimer's disease	90%
Frontotemporal dementia	10%
Huntington's disease	0%

Differential diagnosis of dementias can be difficult, as all are characterized by the core symptom of memory impairment. However, it may be possible to distinguish dementias clinically through other presenting symptoms.

A – Correct. In addition to memory impairment, Alzheimer's disease consists of deficits in language (aphasia), motor function (apraxia), recognition (agnosia), or executive functioning, all of which this patient exhibits. Definitive diagnosis, however, is not possible until autopsy.

B – Incorrect. In frontotemporal dementia, patients often are disinhibited and may be extremely talkative, symptoms that are also not part of this patient's presentation.

C – Incorrect. Huntington's disease is associated with spasmodic movements and incoordination, which are also absent in this patient.

References

Stahl SM. *Stahl's essential psychopharmacology*, fifth edition. New York, NY: Cambridge University Press; 2021. (Chapter 12)

Stahl SM, Morrissette DA. *Stahl's illustrated Alzheimer's disease and other dementias*. New York, NY: Cambridge University Press; 2018.

QUESTION TWO

A medical student with a family history of Alzheimer's disease is interested in learning more about the brain regions involved in memory and the development of Alzheimer's disease. You describe the pathways of acetylcholine, an important neurotransmitter involved in dementia. As part of your explanation, you tell him that major cholinergic projections stemming from the _____ to the _____ are believed to be involved in memory.

A. Striatum; prefrontal cortex

B. Striatum; hypothalamus

C. Basal forebrain; nucleus accumbens

D. Basal forebrain; hippocampus

Dementia and Its Treatment

Answer to Question Two

The correct answer is D.

Choice	Peer answers
Striatum; prefrontal cortex	17%
Striatum; hypothalamus	9%
Basal forebrain; nucleus accumbens	7%
Basal forebrain; hippocampus	67%

A, B, and C – Incorrect.

D – Correct. Acetylcholine is an important neurotransmitter and is thought to be involved in memory. Major acetylcholine neurotransmitter projections originating in the basal forebrain project to the prefrontal cortex, amygdala, and hippocampus, the primary brain structure involved in short-term memory and most greatly affected in Alzheimer's disease.

References

Stahl SM. *Stahl's essential psychopharmacology*, fifth edition. New York, NY: Cambridge University Press; 2021. (Chapter 12)

Woolf NJ, Butcher LL. Cholinergic systems mediate action from movement to higher consciousness. *Behav Brain Res* 2011;221(2):488–98.

Dementia and Its Treatment

QUESTION THREE

A middle-aged man brings his 72-year-old mother in for an appointment because he is concerned that his mother may have Alzheimer's disease. The mother does not feel that anything is wrong, but her son states that she seems somewhat depressed and forgetful lately. Data have shown that:

A. Depression is often comorbid with Alzheimer's disease

B. Depression may increase the risk of developing Alzheimer's disease

C. Depression may be a prodromal symptom of Alzheimer's disease

D. All of the above

E. None of the above

Answer to Question Three

The correct answer is D.

Choice	Peer answers
Depression is often comorbid with Alzheimer's disease	4%
Depression may increase the risk of developing Alzheimer's disease	1%
Depression may be a prodromal symptom of Alzheimer's disease	5%
All of the above	89%
None of the above	1%

A – Partially correct. Mood symptoms can occur as part of Alzheimer's disease and in fact are typically the first notable symptom (often manifested as apathy rather than sadness). In addition, depression is a common comorbid illness in patients with Alzheimer's disease.

B – Partially correct. Depression has been hypothesized to be a possible risk factor for Alzheimer's disease.

C – Partially correct. Depression has been hypothesized to be a possible prodromal symptom of Alzheimer's disease, with some evidence suggesting that it may exacerbate the progression of Alzheimer's pathology.

D – Correct. All of the above.

E – Incorrect (none of the above).

References

Barnes DE, Yaffe K, Byers AL et al. Midlife versus late-life depressive symptoms and risk of dementia: differential effects for Alzheimer's disease and vascular dementia. *Arch Gen Psychiatry* 2012;69(5):493–8.

Pomara N, Bruno D, Sarreal AS et al. Lower CSF amyloid beta peptides and higher F2-isoprostanes in cognitively intact elderly individuals with major depressive disorder. *Am J Psychiatry* 2012;169:523–30.

Stahl SM, Morrissette DA. *Stahl's illustrated Alzheimer's disease and other dementias*. New York, NY: Cambridge University Press; 2018.

Dementia and Its Treatment

QUESTION FOUR

Thomas is a 60-year-old man with a family history of Alzheimer's disease. As a voluntary participant in research studies on Alzheimer's disease, Thomas recently had amyloid positron emission tomography (amyloid PET) neuroimaging done. Although he currently exhibits no behavioral symptoms of Alzheimer's disease, Thomas's amyloid PET scans reveal accumulation of beta amyloid protein throughout cortical and limbic areas of his brain. Although much research is yet to be done, data indicate that the normal physiological role of amyloid beta protein may include:

A. Blood vessel repair functions

B. Antimicrobial functions

C. Both of the above

D. None of the above

Answer to Question Four

The correct answer is C.

Choice	Peer answers
Blood vessel repair functions	17%
Antimicrobial functions	3%
Both of the above	66%
None of the above	14%

A – Partially correct. One hypothesis posits that amyloid beta may act as a sealant at sites of injury or leakage on vessel walls. In this way, amyloid beta may protect from acute brain injury; however, the accumulation of amyloid is associated with development of dementia.

B – Partially correct. Evidence indicates that amyloid beta may have antimicrobial functions. During microbial infection, adhesion of microbes to the host cell is mediated by carbohydrates found in the microbial cell wall. Amyloid beta oligomers bind to cell wall microbial carbohydrates, preventing microbes from adhering to the host cell. This binding of amyloid beta to the microbial cell wall also induces fibrillization of amyloid beta, encompassing microbes and causing agglutination (clumping of microbes so that they can be more readily removed by phagocytosis).

C – Correct. Both blood vessel repair and antimicrobial actions are hypothesized to be normal physiological roles for amyloid beta protein.

D – Incorrect.

References

Atwood CS, Bishop GM, Perry G et al. Amyloid beta: a vascular sealant that protects against hemorrhage? *J Neurosci Res* 2002;70(3):356.

Kokjohn TA, Maarfouf CL, Roher AE. Is Alzheimer's disease amyloidosis the result of a repair mechanism gone astray? *Alzheimers Dement* 2012;8(6):574–83.

Kumar DK, Choi SH, Washicosky KJ et al. Amyloid-beta peptide protects against microbial infection in mouse and worm models of Alzheimer's disease. *Sci Transl Med* 2016;8(340):340ra72.

Stahl SM, Morrissette DA. *Stahl's illustrated Alzheimer's disease and other dementias*. New York, NY: Cambridge University Press; 2018.

QUESTION FIVE

A 68-year-old patient with an early diagnosis of Alzheimer's disease is put on a cholinesterase inhibitor in hopes of improving his cognitive function. This patient has been a chain smoker for over 40 years and refuses to give up the habit. Which of the following medications would *not* be appropriate for this patient, given his smoking habit?

A. Donepezil

B. Galantamine

C. Rivastigmine

D. None of these medications should be prescribed to a patient who smokes

E. There are no contraindications due to smoking for these medications

Answer to Question Five

The correct answer is E.

Choice	Peer answers
Donepezil	12%
Galantamine	9%
Rivastigmine	12%
None of these medications should be prescribed to a patient who smokes	22%
There are no contraindications due to smoking for these medications	45%

A – Incorrect. Donepezil, a reversible, long-acting selective inhibitor of acetylcholinesterase (AChE), may be a good choice, resulting in mainly transient gastrointestinal side effects.

B – Incorrect. Galantamine has a dual mechanism of action: AChE inhibition and positive allosteric modulation (PAM) of nicotinic cholinergic receptors. This may be a good choice for this patient.

C – Incorrect. Rivastigmine, delivered both orally and via a transdermal formulation, has similar safety and efficacy to donepezil. The oral formulation may result in more gastrointestinal side effects than donepezil, owing to its pharmacokinetic profile and inhibition of both AChE and butyrylcholinesterase (BuChE) in the periphery.

D – Incorrect.

E – Correct. One can potentially choose any cholinesterase inhibitor as a first-line treatment since specific contraindications due to smoking do not presently appear in the literature.

References

Stahl SM. *Stahl's essential psychopharmacology, the prescriber's guide*, seventh edition. New York, NY: Cambridge University Press; 2020.

Stahl SM. *Stahl's essential psychopharmacology*, fifth edition. New York, NY: Cambridge University Press; 2021. (Chapter 12)

Dementia and Its Treatment

QUESTION SIX

Marie, a 70-year-old mid-stage Alzheimer's patient, has been on donepezil, 10 mg/day for approximately 8 months to aid in stabilizing her cognitive functioning. Her daughter has noticed a loss of effectiveness over the past month, and they present today to determine a new course of action. You decide to augment Marie's donepezil with 5 mg/day of memantine. Which of the following properties of memantine may be useful in treating Alzheimer's disease?

A. Sigma antagonism

B. Serotonin 3 (5HT3) antagonism

C. N-methyl-D-aspartate (NMDA) antagonism

Dementia and Its Treatment

Answer to Question Six

The correct answer is C.

Choice	Peer answers
Sigma antagonism	3%
Serotonin 3 (5HT3) antagonism	10%
N-methyl-D-aspartate (NMDA) antagonism	88%

A and B – Incorrect. Memantine possesses weak 5HT3 antagonist properties and sigma antagonist properties, but it is currently unclear if these contribute to its benefit in Alzheimer's disease.

C – Correct. Memantine is an NMDA antagonist that binds to the magnesium site. It works as an uncompetitive open channel NMDA receptor antagonist (i.e., low–moderate affinity, voltage dependence, fast-blocking/unblocking kinetics). Memantine is quickly reversible if phasic bursts of glutamate occur but is able to block tonic glutamate release from having negative downstream effects. This hypothetically stops the excessive glutamate from interfering with the resting glutamate neuron's physiological activity, thus improving memory.

References

Kotermanski SE, Johnson JW. Mg^{2+} imparts NMDA receptor subtype selectivity to the Alzheimer's drug memantine. *J Neurosci* 2009;29(9):2774–9.

Stahl SM. *Stahl's essential psychopharmacology*, fifth edition. New York, NY: Cambridge University Press; 2021. (Chapter 12)

Stahl SM, Morrissette DA. *Stahl's illustrated Alzheimer's disease and other dementias*. New York, NY: Cambridge University Press; 2018.

QUESTION SEVEN

Mildred is a 66-year-old patient. She is currently showing no signs of Alzheimer's disease but is considering enrolling in one of the ongoing Alzheimer's disease immunotherapy-based clinical trials. You explain to Mildred that such immunotherapy involves:

A. Antibodies that bind to NMDA receptors

B. Antibodies that bind to amyloid protein

C. Antibodies that bind to tau protein

D. B and C

Answer to Question Seven

The correct answer is D.

Choice	Peer answers
Antibodies that bind to NMDA receptors	4%
Antibodies that bind to amyloid protein	11%
Antibodies that bind to tau protein	1%
B and C	83%

A – Incorrect. Although the currently available Alzheimer's drug memantine acts by antagonizing NMDA receptors, the ongoing immunotherapy clinical trials do not involve antibodies that bind to NMDA receptors.

B – Partially correct. Many ongoing immunotherapy clinical trials utilize various antibodies that bind to different portions or conformations of the amyloid beta peptide and are thought to remove amyloid beta from the brain via three hypothesized mechanisms. These mechanisms include: peripheral sink, disaggregation, and microglia engagement and phagocytosis.

C – Partially correct. Given that numerous immunotherapy trials utilizing antibodies that bind to amyloid beta have yielded less than satisfactory results, there are now several clinical trials involving tau immunotherapy that are underway.

D – Correct.

References

Alzheimer's Association. 2016 Alzheimer's disease facts and figures. *Alzheimers Dement* 2016;12(4):459–509.

Godyń J, Jończyk J, Panek D et al. Therapeutic strategies for Alzheimer's disease in clinical trials. *Pharmacol Rep* 2016;68:127–38.

Harrison JR, Owen MJ. Alzheimer's disease: the amyloid hypothesis on trial. *Br J Psychiatry* 2016;208(1):1–3.

Panza F, Seripa D, Solfrizzi V et al. Emerging drugs to reduce abnormal β-amyloid protein in Alzheimer's disease patients. *Expert Opin Emerg Drugs* 2016;21(4):377–91.

Pedersen JT, Sigurdsson EM. Tau immunotherapy for Alzheimer's disease. *Trends Mol Med* 2015;21(6):394–402.

QUESTION EIGHT

Diane is a 66-year-old patient with a family history of dementia. Genotyping of this patient reveals a mutation in her gene for amyloid precursor protein (APP). Which APP mutation is *not* associated with increased development of familial Alzheimer's disease?

A. Flemish mutation

B. Icelandic mutation

C. London mutation

D. Swedish mutation

Answer to Question Eight

The correct answer is B.

Choice	Peer answers
Flemish mutation	17%
Icelandic mutation	50%
London mutation	20%
Swedish mutation	13%

A and C – Incorrect. The Flemish and London mutations both affect processing of APP by gamma-secretase leading to increased production of beta amyloid. Both mutations are associated with increased development of familial Alzheimer's disease.

B – Correct. The Icelandic mutation on the APP gene actually *reduces* the cleavage of APP by the beta-secretase enzyme, resulting in decreased beta amyloid production and decreasing risk of developing familial Alzheimer's disease.

D – Incorrect. The Swedish mutation leads to increased cleavage of APP by the beta-secretase enzyme, leading to increased beta amyloid production and increased development of familial Alzheimer's disease.

References
Giri M, Zhang M, Lu Y. Genes associated with Alzheimer's disease: an overview and current status. *Clin Interv Aging* 2016;11:665–81.

Hinz FI, Geschwind DH. Molecular genetics of neurodegenerative dementias. *Cold Spring Harb Perspect Biol* 2017;9(4):a023705.

Rosenberg RN, Lambracht-Washington D, Yu G et al. Genomics of Alzheimer disease: a review. *JAMA Neurol* 2016;73(7):867–74.

Schellenberg GD, Montine TJ. The genetics and neuropathology of Alzheimer's disease. *Acta Neuropathol* 2012;124(3):305–23.

Dementia and Its Treatment

QUESTION NINE

A 79-year-old man presents to your office with his wife. She lists significant medical history, such as chronic renal failure, mild cirrhosis, arrhythmia, and a recent diagnosis of moderately severe Alzheimer's disease by their family physician. Which of the following medications for Alzheimer's disease has a "do not use" warning for patients with renal and hepatic impairment?

A. Rivastigmine

B. Memantine

C. Galantamine

D. Donepezil

Answer to Question Nine

The correct answer is C.

Choice	Peer answers
Rivastigmine	21%
Memantine	15%
Galantamine	45%
Donepezil	19%

A – Incorrect. Rivastigmine, a cholinesterase inhibitor, appears as though it could be useful in this situation, as it can be used in patients with renal or hepatic impairment; caution should be exercised in cardiac patients due to potential syncopal episodes.

B – Incorrect. Memantine, an NMDA receptor antagonist, would be useful in this case due to its indication of approval for treatment of moderate to severe dementia, with which this patient has been diagnosed, although the label indicates a lowered dose for use in severe renal impairment. However, there is not likely to be a problem for hepatic or cardiac impaired patients.

C – Correct. Galantamine has a "do not use" warning in patients with renal and hepatic impairment, as well as a caution warning when used in cardiac impaired patients. Furthermore, galantamine, a cholinesterase inhibitor, is often prescribed as one of the first-line treatments for early-stage Alzheimer's, rather than moderately severe cases.

D – Incorrect. Donepezil, a cholinesterase inhibitor, could potentially be given to this patient to aid in treatment of Alzheimer's, though little data has been gathered on its effects regarding renal and hepatic impairment. Cardiac patients should use this drug with caution due to reports of syncopal episodes.

Reference
Stahl SM, Morrissette DA. *Stahl's illustrated Alzheimer's disease and other dementias*. New York, NY: Cambridge University Press; 2018.

QUESTION TEN

Virgil is a 65-year-old man. His daughter reports that he began forgetting birthdays, grandchildren's names, and other important information approximately 1 year ago and that he has become increasingly unable to perform many activities, such as paying bills on time. Neuropsychiatric testing shows moderate cognitive impairment not attributable to any medical or psychiatric condition. Virgil has never been tested for biomarkers of Alzheimer's disease, but genetic testing has revealed that he carries an Alzheimer's-associated mutation in the presenilin gene. What would be the most likely diagnosis for this patient according to the National Institute on Aging and Alzheimer's Association 2011 diagnostic criteria for dementia?

A. Possible Alzheimer's dementia

B. Probable Alzheimer's dementia with increased level of certainty

C. Alzheimer's dementia

Answer to Question Ten

The correct answer is B.

Choice	Peer answers
Possible Alzheimer's dementia	9%
Probable Alzheimer's dementia with increased level of certainty	73%
Alzheimer's dementia	18%

A – Incorrect. The diagnosis of "possible Alzheimer's dementia" is reserved for individuals who exhibit dementia with an atypical course and mixed presentation, which is not demonstrated in this patient's case. In instances where the dementia is atypical or mixed in its presentation, and especially without biomarker evidence, such dementia could be due to Alzheimer's disease, Lewy body dementia, vascular dementia, or frontotemporal dementia (or some combination of the pathologies associated with each of these dementia types).

B – Correct. This patient is exhibiting the typical symptoms of Alzheimer's dementia including an insidious onset, with a history of worsening cognition, amnesic symptoms, and deficits in executive function being the most prominent symptoms. Although biomarker evidence (including positive amyloid PET neuroimaging and increased cerebrospinal fluid tau levels) would increase the certainty of the diagnosis, the fact that this patient carries the Alzheimer's disease-associated presenilin mutation allows us to make the diagnosis of "probable Alzheimer's dementia with increased level of certainty."

C – Incorrect. The only way to currently make a confirmed diagnosis of Alzheimer's dementia is through postmortem visualization of Alzheimer's neuropathology.

Reference

McKhann GM, Knopman DS, Chertkow H et al. The diagnosis of dementia due to Alzheimer's disease: recommendations from the National Institute on Aging-Alzheimer's Association workgroups on diagnostic guidelines for Alzheimer's disease. *Alzheimers Dement* 2011;7(3):263–9.

Dementia and Its Treatment

QUESTION ELEVEN

Ellie is a 59-year-old patient who presents with hypoglycemia. She also presents with symptoms that could be either dementia or delirium. One key feature that can help differentiate delirium from dementia is:

A. Psychosis

B. Memory deficits

C. Disorientation

D. Acute and fluctuating course

Answer to Question Eleven

The correct answer is D.

Choice	Peer answers
Psychosis	4%
Memory deficits	3%
Disorientation	2%
Acute and fluctuating course	92%

A, B, and C – Incorrect. Both dementia and delirium may present clinically with memory deficits, disorientation, and psychosis as well as impaired judgment and confusion.

D – Correct. The presentation of delirium is usually acute and fluctuating whereas dementia is typically a chronic condition that does not fluctuate. Delirium also typically involves cloudiness of consciousness, and sleep disturbances compared to dementia.

References

Ford AH. Preventing delirium in dementia: managing risk factors. *Maturitas* 2016;92:35–40.

Lippmann S, **Perugula ML**. Delirium or dementia? *Innov Clin Neurosci* 2016;13(9–10):56–7.

QUESTION TWELVE

A 75-year-old patient with mild cognitive impairment is suspected of being in the early, prodromal stage of Alzheimer's disease. Which biomarker evidence would support a diagnosis of Alzheimer's disease?

A. Decreased cerebrospinal fluid (CSF) levels of amyloid beta

B. Increased CSF levels of tau protein

C. Increased levels of brain amyloid beta on PET scans

D. All of the above

Answer to Question Twelve

The correct answer is D.

Choice	Peer answers
Decreased cerebrospinal fluid (CSF) levels of amyloid beta	2%
Increased CSF levels of tau protein	3%
Increased levels of brain amyloid beta on PET scans	9%
All of the above	85%

A – Partially correct. During the presymptomatic stage of Alzheimer's disease, amyloid-beta peptides are slowly and relentlessly deposited into the brain rather than eliminated via the CSF, plasma, and liver. Therefore, CSF levels of amyloid beta actually decrease.

B – Partially correct. As Alzheimer's disease progresses, tau and phosphorylated tau protein levels in the CSF increase.

C – Partially correct. Levels of brain amyloid beta can be detected with PET scans using radioactive neuroimaging tracers that bind to the fibrillar form of amyloid and thus label mature neuritic plaques. In normal controls, amyloid PET imaging typically shows the absence of amyloid. However, individuals who are cognitively normal may have moderate accumulation of amyloid; these individuals may be in the presymptomatic first stage of Alzheimer's disease. In the final stage of Alzheimer's disease, when full-blown dementia is clinically evident, a large accumulation of brain amyloid can readily be seen.

D – Correct.

Reference
Stahl SM, Morrissette DA. *Stahl's illustrated Alzheimer's disease and other dementias*. New York, NY: Cambridge University Press; 2018.

QUESTION THIRTEEN

William is a 77-year-old patient with mid- to late-stage Alzheimer's disease. His behavioral impairment has drastically worsened over the past month. The patient's family is concerned that William's rapidly deteriorating psychiatric and physical functioning may be due to his medication (donepezil 10 mg/day) no longer working. The treating clinician feels that Alzheimer's disease may not be the primary cause of William's recent deterioration. Which comorbid illness most commonly goes undetected in patients with moderate to severe dementia?

A. Bacteriuria

B. Dehydration

C. Hypothyroidism

Dementia and Its Treatment

STAHL'S SELF-ASSESSMENT EXAMINATION IN PSYCHIATRY

Answer to Question Thirteen

The correct answer is A.

Choice	Peer answers
Bacteriuria	71%
Dehydration	20%
Hypothyroidism	9%

A – Correct. Nearly 40% of individuals with dementia may be suffering from an undetected but modifiable illness. Bacteriuria is the most common undiagnosed illness in patients suffering from dementia, and it can lead to incontinence and increased agitation.

B – Incorrect. Although untreated dehydration has been found in 3% of individuals with dementia, it is not the most common undetected comorbid illness.

C – Incorrect. Although untreated hypothyroidism has been found in 1–3% of individuals with dementia, it is not the most common undetected comorbid illness.

Reference

Hodgson NA, Gitlin LN, Winter L et al. Undiagnosed illness and neuropsychiatric behaviors in community residing older adults with dementia. *Alzheimer Dis Assoc Disord* 2011;25:109–15.

QUESTION FOURTEEN

Mitchell is a 90-year-old patient with Lewy body dementia. His daughter, who is his full-time caregiver, reports that her father has started to exhibit worsening of agitation, wandering, and confusion in the early evening – also known as sundowning. Which of the following treatments has actually been shown to worsen sundowning behavior?

A. Melatonin

B. Cholinesterase inhibitors

C. Bright light therapy

D. Benzodiazepines

Dementia and Its Treatment

Answer to Question Fourteen

The correct answer is D.

Choice	Peer answers
Melatonin	6%
Cholinesterase inhibitors	7%
Bright light therapy	3%
Benzodiazepines	84%

A, B, and C – Incorrect. There is some, albeit limited, evidence that bright light therapy, cholinesterase inhibitors (specifically donepezil), and melatonin may improve sundowning behavior.

D – Correct. The use of benzodiazepines and other hypnotics has been linked with a paradoxical increase in behavioral issues, such as sundowning, in patients with dementia. Furthermore, benzodiazepines are particularly not recommended in elderly patients with dementia as they may greatly increase the risk of falls, fractures, and death as well as worsening cognitive impairment.

References

Canevelli M, Valleta M, Trebbastoni A et al. Sundowning in dementia: clinical relevance, pathophysiological determinants, and therapeutic approaches. *Front Med (Lausanne)* 2016;3:73.

Satlin A, Volicer L, Ross V et al. Bright light treatment of behavioral and sleep disturbances in patients with Alzheimer's disease. *Am J Psychiatry* 1992;149(8):1028–32.

Skjerve A, Nygaard HA. Improvement in sundowning in dementia with Lewy bodies after treatment with donepezil. *Int J Geriatr Psychiatry* 2000;15(12):1147–51.

Stahl SM, Morrissette DA. *Stahl's illustrated Alzheimer's disease and other dementias*. New York, NY: Cambridge University Press; 2018.

CHAPTER PEER COMPARISON

For the Dementia section, the correct answer was selected 72% of the time.

7 PSYCHOSIS AND ITS TREATMENT

QUESTION ONE

A 24-year-old male initially presents with acute auditory hallu-cinations and is treated with medication. Four days later he arrives at your office for evaluation. You observe that he is neatly dressed, avoids eye contact, and gives very short answers to your initial questions. Which of the following questions would be most bene-ficial for determining his degree of negative symptoms?

A. How often have you visited with friends in the past week?

B. Have the voices you've heard persisted or returned?

C. Have you ever thought about hurting yourself or someone else?

D. In the past week have you had difficulty concentrating?

Answer to Question One

The correct answer is A.

Choice	Peer answers
How often have you visited with friends in the past week?	77%
Have the voices you've heard persisted or returned?	6%
Have you ever thought about hurting yourself or someone else?	6%
In the past week have you had difficulty concentrating?	11%

A – Correct. How often have you visited with friends in the past week? This is a useful question when assessing for negative symptoms, as an important component of negative symptoms is reduced social drive.

B – Incorrect. Have the voices you've heard persisted or returned? Although this question is useful for determining the presence of positive symptoms, it is not applicable to assessment of negative symptoms.

C – Incorrect. Have you ever thought about hurting yourself or someone else? This question can help assess for risk of suicide as well as any possible aggression risk, but these are not part of the negative symptom domain.

D – Incorrect. In the past week have you had difficulty concentrating? This question is applicable to assessment for cognitive symptoms, but not for negative symptoms.

References

Stahl SM. *Stahl's essential psychopharmacology*, fifth edition. New York, NY: Cambridge University Press; 2021. (Chapter 4)

Stahl SM, Buckley PF. Negative symptoms of schizophrenia: a problem that will not go away. *Acta Psychiatr Scand* 2007;15:4–11.

QUESTION TWO

A 21-year-old man who has just been diagnosed with schizophrenia presents with his parents. He speaks with a reserved and simple language-processing style; he is able to understand and relate to simple questions but seems to get lost when the pace of the conversation between the clinician and parents accelerates. When reviewing the patient's history, what pattern of cognitive functioning prior to psychosis onset would you be most likely to find?

A. Normal cognitive functioning during premorbid and prodromal phases

B. Impaired cognitive functioning that is stable across premorbid and prodromal phases

C. Impaired cognitive functioning premorbidly with further decline during the prodromal phase

D. Progressive decline of cognitive functioning premorbidly, which stabilizes in the prodromal phase

Psychosis and Its Treatment

Answer to Question Two

The correct answer is C.

Choice	Peer answers
Normal cognitive functioning during premorbid and prodromal phases	8%
Impaired cognitive functioning that is stable across premorbid and prodromal phases	6%
Impaired cognitive functioning premorbidly with further decline during the prodromal phase	76%
Progressive decline of cognitive functioning premorbidly, which stabilizes in the prodromal phase	11%

Individuals who ultimately develop schizophrenia typically exhibit a deficit in cognitive and social functioning that **begins in childhood**, with a **notable decline** in cognitive and social functioning that occurs during adolescence and precedes the onset of psychosis. This decline in cognitive functioning coincides with the neurodevelopmental period known as competitive elimination, during which extensive brain restructuring and synaptic pruning takes place.

A – Incorrect. Individuals with schizophrenia typically exhibit a history of cognitive impairment prior to psychosis onset.

B – Incorrect. Individuals with schizophrenia typically experience a decline in functioning during the prodromal phase.

C – Correct. Individuals with schizophrenia typically exhibit impaired cognitive functioning premorbidly with a notable decline during the prodromal phase.

D – Incorrect. Individuals with schizophrenia generally show stable cognitive functioning premorbidly, with decline not occurring until the prodromal phase.

References
Insel TR. Rethinking schizophrenia. *Nature* 2010;468:187–93.

McGorry PD, Yung AR, Bechdolf A, Amminger P. Back to the future: predicting and reshaping the course of psychotic disorder. *Arch Gen Psychiatry* 2008;65:25–7.

QUESTION THREE

A 24-year-old woman is hospitalized after an altercation in which she screamed at and attacked her neighbor when he knocked on her door. Her mother reports that she has been increasingly erratic recently, with emotional outbursts and impulsive behavior. Which of the following brain regions is most likely associated with these symptoms?

A. Dorsolateral prefrontal cortex

B. Nucleus accumbens

C. Orbital frontal cortex

D. Substantia nigra

Answer to Question Three

The correct answer is C.

Choice	Peer answers
Dorsolateral prefrontal cortex	32%
Nucleus accumbens	9%
Orbital frontal cortex	54%
Substantia nigra	5%

A – Incorrect. Dorsolateral prefrontal cortex: this brain region is hypothetically associated with cognition and executive functioning, not with aggression.

B – Incorrect. Nucleus accumbens: this brain region is hypothetically associated with positive symptoms such as delusions and hallucinations. Although aggressive symptoms, such as those exhibited by this patient, often occur in conjunction with positive symptoms, they may not be localized to the nucleus accumbens.

C – Correct. Orbital frontal cortex: aggressive symptoms such as those exhibited by this patient are hypothetically associated with impairment in impulse control, which is largely regulated by the orbital frontal cortex.

D – Incorrect. Substantia nigra: this region in the brainstem houses dopaminergic cell bodies that project to the striatum. The substantia nigra is not particularly linked to aggression.

Reference
Stahl SM. *Stahl's essential psychopharmacology*, fifth edition. New York, NY: Cambridge University Press; 2021. (Chapter 4)

QUESTION FOUR

A major current hypothesis for the cause of schizophrenia proposes that *N*-methyl-D-aspartate (NMDA) receptors may be:

A. Hypofunctional

B. Hyperfunctional

Answer to Question Four

The correct answer is A.

Choice	Peer answers
Hypofunctional	69%
Hyperfunctional	31%

A – Correct. A major current hypothesis for the cause of schizophrenia proposes that glutamate activity at NMDA receptors is hypofunctional due to abnormalities in the formation of glutamatergic NMDA synapses during neurodevelopment.

Normally, when glutamate synapses are active, their NMDA receptors trigger an electrical phenomenon known as long-term potentiation, or LTP. LTP leads to structural and functional changes of the synapse that make neurotransmission more efficient, sometimes called "strengthening" of synapses. During pubescence and adolescence, a period known as competitive elimination occurs, with extensive synaptic pruning and restructuring. Frequently used synaptic connections with efficient NMDA neurotransmission survive, whereas infrequently used synaptic connections with less active NMDA receptors may be targets for elimination. This shaping of the brain's circuits normally allows the most critical synapses to survive, while inefficient and rarely utilized synapses are eliminated. Abnormalities in the NMDA receptor may jeopardize this essential process and increase risk for neurodevelopmental disorders such as schizophrenia.

B – Incorrect. NMDA receptors are not hypothesized to be hyperfunctional in schizophrenia.

Reference
Stahl SM. *Stahl's essential psychopharmacology*, fifth edition. New York, NY: Cambridge University Press; 2021. (Chapter 4)

QUESTION FIVE

According to the dopamine hypothesis of schizophrenia, which underlying neurobiological mechanisms are associated with positive symptoms?

A. Hyperactive mesocortical dopamine pathway to the dorsolateral prefrontal cortex (DLPFC) and ventromedial prefrontal cortex (VMPFC)

B. Hyperactive mesolimbic pathway

C. Hypoactive mesocortical dopamine pathway to the DLPFC and VMPFC

D. Hypoactive mesolimbic pathway

Answer to Question Five

The correct answer is B.

Choice	Peer answers
Hyperactive mesocortical dopamine pathway to the dorsolateral prefrontal cortex (DLPFC) and ventromedial prefrontal cortex (VMPFC)	28%
Hyperactive mesolimbic pathway	61%
Hypoactive mesocortical dopamine pathway to the DLPFC and VMPFC	9%
Hypoactive mesolimbic pathway	2%

A – Incorrect. In untreated schizophrenia, the mesocortical dopamine pathways to the DLPFC and to the VMPFC are hypothesized to be hypoactive. This hypoactivity is related to cognitive symptoms (in the DLPFC), negative symptoms (in the DLPFC and VMPFC), and affective symptoms of schizophrenia (in the VMPFC). These pathways are not associated with positive symptoms.

B – Correct. In untreated schizophrenia, the mesolimbic pathway is hypothesized to be hyperactive, resulting in excess dopamine at the synapse, which leads to positive symptoms such as delusions and hallucinations.

C – Incorrect.

D – Incorrect.

Reference
Stahl SM. *Stahl's essential psychopharmacology*, fifth edition. New York, NY: Cambridge University Press; 2021. (Chapter 5)

QUESTION SIX

Tim is a 17-year-old patient with first-onset schizophrenia. He is currently taking the antipsychotic fluphenazine but is not experiencing any relief from his positive symptoms. Lab testing reveals that Tim's fluphenazine plasma levels are low; thus, there may not be sufficient blockade of dopamine D2 receptors. In order for an antipsychotic to exert therapeutic effects, what is the minimum hypothetical threshold of D2 receptor occupancy?

A. >20%

B. >40%

C. >60%

D. >90%

Answer to Question Six

The correct answer is C.

Choice	Peer answers
>20%	2%
>40%	16%
>60%	79%
>90%	3%

A – Incorrect. With only 20% D2 receptor occupancy, it is unlikely that a pharmacological agent will have any therapeutic effects.

B – Incorrect. With only 40% D2 receptor occupancy, it is unlikely that a pharmacological agent will have any therapeutic effects.

C – Correct. Data indicate that 60% D2 receptor occupancy is the minimum threshold for antipsychotic efficacy.

D – Incorrect. D2 receptor occupancy of 90% is well above the hypothetical minimum threshold for antipsychotic effects and is also above the hypothetical threshold for inducing drug-induced parkinsonism.

Reference

Morrisette DM, Stahl SM. Treating the violent patient with psychosis or impulsivity utilizing antipsychotic polypharmacy and high-dose monotherapy. *CNS Spectr* 2014;19(5):439–48.

QUESTION SEVEN

Based on thorough evaluation of a patient and his history, his care provider intends to begin treatment with a conventional antipsychotic but has not selected a particular agent yet. Which of the following is most true about conventional antipsychotics?

A. They are very similar in therapeutic profile but differ in side effect profile

B. They are very similar in both therapeutic and side effect profile

C. They differ in therapeutic profile but are similar in side effect profile

D. They differ in both therapeutic and side effect profile

Answer to Question Seven

The correct answer is A.

Choice	Peer answers
They are very similar in therapeutic profile but differ in side effect profile	66%
They are very similar in both therapeutic and side effect profile	17%
They differ in therapeutic profile but are similar in side effect profile	7%
They differ in both therapeutic and side effect profile	11%

A – Correct. Although individual effects may vary from patient to patient, in general conventional antipsychotics share the same primary mechanism of action and do not differ much in their therapeutic profiles. There are, however, differences in secondary properties, such as degree of muscarinic, histaminergic, and/or alpha-adrenergic receptor antagonism, which can lead to different side effect profiles.

B, C, and D – Incorrect.

References
Stahl SM. *Essential psychopharmacology, the prescriber's guide*, seventh edition. New York, NY: Cambridge University Press; 2020.

Stahl SM. *Stahl's essential psychopharmacology*, fifth edition. New York, NY: Cambridge University Press; 2021. (Chapter 5)

QUESTION EIGHT

A 34-year-old man is initiated on an atypical antipsychotic for the treatment of schizophrenia. The majority of atypical antipsychotics:

A. Have higher affinity for dopamine 2 receptors than for serotonin 2A receptors

B. Have higher affinity for serotonin 2A receptors than for dopamine 2 receptors

C. Don't have affinity for dopamine 2 receptors or serotonin 2A receptors

Psychosis and Its Treatment

STAHL'S SELF-ASSESSMENT EXAMINATION IN PSYCHIATRY

Answer to Question Eight

The correct answer is B.

Choice	Peer answers
Have higher affinity for dopamine 2 receptors than for serotonin 2A receptors	32%
Have higher affinity for serotonin 2A receptors than for dopamine 2 receptors	68%
Don't have affinity for dopamine 2 receptors or serotonin 2A receptors	1%

A – Incorrect. Nearly all atypical antipsychotics have an affinity for blocking serotonin 2A receptors that is equal to or greater than their affinity for blocking dopamine 2 receptors.

B – Correct. Serotonin neurons originate in the raphe nucleus of the brainstem and project throughout the brain, including to the cortex. They synapse there with glutamatergic pyramidal neurons, which project to the substantia nigra in the brainstem. The substantia nigra is the origin of dopaminergic neurons that project to the striatum. All serotonin 2A receptors are postsynaptic. When they are located on cortical pyramidal neurons, they are excitatory. Thus, when serotonin is released in the cortex and binds to serotonin 2A receptors on glutamatergic pyramidal neurons, this stimulates them to release glutamate in the brainstem, which in turn stimulates gamma-aminobutyric acid (GABA) release. GABA binds to dopaminergic neurons projecting from the substantia nigra to the striatum, inhibiting dopamine release.

Nearly all atypical antipsychotics have an affinity for blocking serotonin 2A receptors that is equal to or greater than their affinity for blocking dopamine 2 receptors. The "pines" – clozapine, olanzapine, quetiapine, asenapine, and zotepine – all bind much more potently to the serotonin 2A receptor than they do to the dopamine 2 receptor. The "dones" and "rone" – risperidone, paliperidone, ziprasidone, iloperidone, lurasidone, and lumateperone – also bind more potently to the serotonin 2A receptor than to the dopamine 2 receptor or show similar potency at both receptors. Aripiprazole and cariprazine bind more potently to the dopamine 2 receptor than to the serotonin 2A receptor; however, they are also partial agonists at dopamine 2 receptors. Brexpiprazole (also a dopamine 2 partial agonist) has comparable binding affinity to the dopamine 2 and serotonin 2A receptors.

C – Incorrect.

Psychosis and Its Treatment

References

Roth BL. Ki determinations, receptor binding profiles, agonist and/or antagonist functional data, HERG data, MDR1 data, etc. as appropriate was generously provided by the National Institute of Mental Health's Psychoactive Drug Screening Program, Contract # HHSN-271–2008–00025-C (NIMH PDSP). The NIMH PDSP is directed by Bryan L. Roth, MD, PhD at the University of North Carolina at Chapel Hill and Project Officer Jamie Driscol at NIMH, Bethesda, MD, USA. For experimental details please refer to the PDSP website http://pdsp.med.unc.edu.

Stahl SM. *Stahl's essential psychopharmacology*, fifth edition. New York, NY: Cambridge University Press; 2021. (Chapter 5)

QUESTION NINE

A 34-year-old male recently began experiencing breast secretions while receiving perphenazine. After switching to quetiapine, the secretions ceased. Which of the following is the most likely pharmacological explanation for the resolution of this side effect?

A. Dopamine 2 antagonism

B. Serotonin 2A antagonism

C. Serotonin 2C antagonism

D. Histamine 1 antagonism

Answer to Question Nine

The correct answer is B.

Choice	Peer answers
Dopamine 2 antagonism	30%
Serotonin 2A antagonism	54%
Serotonin 2C antagonism	11%
Histamine 1 antagonism	6%

A – Incorrect. Stimulation of dopamine 2 receptors inhibits prolactin release; thus, a dopamine 2 antagonist such as perphenazine could increase prolactin release and potentially lead to breast secretions.

B – Correct. Stimulation of serotonin 2A receptors stimulates prolactin release. Since they have opposing effects on prolactin, adding serotonin 2A antagonism to dopamine 2 antagonism results in a neutral effect on prolactin and may relieve breast secretions caused by dopamine 2 antagonism alone.

C and D – Incorrect. Although quetiapine is an antagonist at serotonin 2C and histamine 1 receptors, both of which are associated with some side effects, neither receptor type has an established role in prolactin elevation.

Reference

Stahl SM. *Stahl's essential psychopharmacology*, fifth edition. New York, NY: Cambridge University Press; 2021. (Chapter 5)

QUESTION TEN

Compared to aripiprazole, where do brexpiprazole and cariprazine fall on the dopamine agonist spectrum?

A. Brexpiprazole and cariprazine have less intrinsic activity/are more antagonistic than aripiprazole

B. Brexpiprazole and cariprazine have more intrinsic activity/are more of an agonist than aripiprazole

C. Brexpiprazole and cariprazine have about the same intrinsic activity/are equally antagonistic compared to aripiprazole

Answer to Question Ten

The correct answer is A.

Choice	Peer answers
Brexpiprazole and cariprazine have less intrinsic activity/are more antagonistic than aripiprazole	52%
Brexpiprazole and cariprazine have more intrinsic activity/are more of an agonist than aripiprazole	29%
Brexpiprazole and cariprazine have about the same intrinsic activity/are equally antagonistic compared to aripiprazole	19%

A – Correct. Brexpiprazole and cariprazine, like aripiprazole, are partial agonists at the dopamine 2 receptor. Pharmacologically, brexpiprazole has less intrinsic activity (i.e., is less of a partial agonist and more of an antagonist) at dopamine 2 receptors than aripiprazole. Similarly, cariprazine also has less intrinsic activity at dopamine 2 receptors than aripiprazole; its activity is very similar to brexpiprazole. Cariprazine and brexpiprazole differ from each other in terms of their secondary pharmacological properties.

B – Incorrect.

C – Incorrect.

References

Stahl SM. Mechanism of action of brexpiprazole: comparison with aripiprazole. *CNS Spectr* 2016;21:1–6.

Stahl SM. Mechanism of action of cariprazine. *CNS Spectr* 2016;21:123–7.

Psychosis and Its Treatment

QUESTION ELEVEN

Frank is a 24-year-old patient recently diagnosed with schizo-phrenia. He is currently taking an antipsychotic, and his psychosis symptoms are reasonably well resolved. At a follow-up visit, you notice that Frank does not seem to be able to sit still; he is con-stantly pacing the examining room, and when he does sit down, he rocks back and forth, fidgets, and repetitively crosses and uncrosses his legs. Drug-induced akathisia is caused by:

A. Dopaminergic hypoactivity

B. Dopaminergic hyperactivity

C. Unknown pathophysiology

Psychosis and Its Treatment

Answer to Question Eleven

The correct answer is C.

Choice	Peer answers
Dopaminergic hypoactivity	28%
Dopaminergic hyperactivity	30%
Unknown pathophysiology	42%

Akathisia is a distressing side effect characterized by a subjective feeling of inner restlessness that prompts a need to move. It is often extraordinarily difficult for the patient to describe, in part because there are few subjective states to which it can be compared.

A – Incorrect. Dopaminergic hypoactivity has been proposed as an underlying cause of akathisia because most antipsychotics are potent antagonists at the dopamine 2 receptor, it occurs in Parkinson's disease, and similar disorders (restless legs syndrome and periodic limb movement disorder) are treated with dopamine agonists. However, there is no established direct link between parkinsonism and akathisia, and agents that cause the least drug-induced parkinsonism can still cause akathisia. In addition, other agents can also cause akathisia, including notably the selective serotonin reuptake inhibitors (SSRIs).

B – Incorrect. Akathisia has not been linked to dopamine hyperactivity.

C – Correct. The pathophysiology of akathisia is not known.

References

Lohr JB, Eidt CA, Abdulrazzaq Alfaraj A, Soliman MA. The clinical challenges of akathisia. *CNS Spectr* 2015;20:4–14.

Stahl SM, Loonen AJ. The mechanism of drug-induced akathisia. *CNS Spectr* 2011;16(1):7–10.

QUESTION TWELVE

A 44-year-old woman with schizophrenia has developed tardive dyskinesia after taking haloperidol 15 mg/day for 2 years. Which of the following would be the most appropriate pharmacological mechanism to manage her tardive dyskinesia?

A. Antagonism at serotonin 2A receptors

B. Antagonism of beta-adrenergic receptors

C. Inhibition of vesicular monoamine transporter 2

D. Antagonism of muscarinic acetylcholine receptors

Psychosis and Its Treatment

Answer to Question Twelve

The correct answer is C.

Choice	Peer answers
Antagonism at serotonin 2A receptors	10%
Antagonism of beta-adrenergic receptors	6%
Inhibition of vesicular monoamine transporter 2	57%
Antagonism of muscarinic acetylcholine receptors	26%

Tardive dyskinesia is a neurological disorder characterized by repetitive involuntary movements usually associated with lower facial and distal extremity musculature. Common signs include tongue protrusion, writhing of tongue, lip smacking, chewing, blinking, and grimacing. Tardive dyskinesia will reverse in approximately one-third of patients over a 6-month period after the offending medication is discontinued. For patients who do not experience reversal of their tardive dyskinesia, there are augmentation options to treat it.

A – Incorrect. Although dopamine 2 antagonists with the additional property of serotonin 2A antagonism were initially thought to carry less risk of tardive dyskinesia, it is now known that tardive dyskinesia continues to be a potential side effect of these agents, and that any possibly reduced risk does not necessarily seem to correlate with the degree of serotonin 2A antagonism.

B – Incorrect. Beta-blockers (e.g., propranolol) do not show evidence of efficacy in the treatment of tardive dyskinesia.

C – Correct. The best evidenced (including approved) medications to treat tardive dyskinesia are selective inhibitors of vesicular monoamine transporter 2 (VMAT2), which packages monoamines, including dopamine, into synaptic vesicles of presynaptic neurons in the central nervous system.

D – Incorrect. Central anticholinergic medication can improve drug-induced parkinsonism but exacerbate or unmask tardive dyskinesia. This effect may be reversible if the anticholinergic medication is discontinued.

References

Fernandez HH, Factor SA, Hauser RA et al. Randomized controlled trial of deutetrabenazine for tardive dyskinesia: the ARM-TD study. *Neurology* 2017;88(21):2003–10.

Psychosis and Its Treatment

Hauser RA, Factor SA, Marder SR et al. KINECT 3: a phase 3
randomized, double-blind, placebo-controlled trial of valbenazine for
tardive dyskinesia. *Am J Psychiatry* 2017;174(5):476–84.

Waln O, Jankovic J. An update on tardive dyskinesia: from
phenomenology to treatment. *Tremor Other Hyperkinet Mov (NY)*
2013;3:tre-03-161-4138-1. doi:10.7916/D88P5Z71.

Psychosis and Its Treatment

QUESTION THIRTEEN

A patient who has been taking an atypical antipsychotic for 6 months has experienced a 22-pound weight gain since baseline. Which of the following pharmacological properties most likely underlies this patient's metabolic changes?

A. Dopamine 2 antagonism

B. Serotonin 2A antagonism

C. Serotonin 2C antagonism

D. Alpha 1 adrenergic antagonism

Answer to Question Thirteen

The correct answer is C.

Choice	Peer answers
Dopamine 2 antagonism	6%
Serotonin 2A antagonism	21%
Serotonin 2C antagonism	65%
Alpha 1 adrenergic antagonism	8%

A – Incorrect. Antagonism of dopamine 2 receptors is associated with both therapeutic and side effects but is not linked to weight gain.

B – Incorrect. Similarly, antagonism of serotonin 2A receptors has not been linked to risk for weight gain.

C – Correct. Antagonism of serotonin 2C receptors is associated with increased risk for weight gain, perhaps in part due to stimulation of appetite regulated by the hypothalamus, and especially in combination with histamine 1 antagonism.

D – Incorrect. Antagonism of alpha 1 adrenergic receptors is associated with side effects but is not linked to weight gain.

References
Stahl SM. *Essential psychopharmacology, the prescriber's guide*, seventh edition. New York, NY: Cambridge University Press; 2020.

Stahl SM. *Stahl's essential psychopharmacology*, fifth edition. New York, NY: Cambridge University Press; 2021. (Chapter 5)

QUESTION FOURTEEN

A 34-year-old woman with schizophrenia has been taking a therapeutic dose of olanzapine (20 mg/day) for 6 weeks. She has shown no response but also exhibits no side effects. The **ideal** course of action at this point would be to:

A. Obtain a plasma level of olanzapine

B. Raise the dose of olanzapine

C. Switch to a different antipsychotic

D. Add a mood-stabilizing anticonvulsant

Answer to Question Fourteen

The correct answer is A.

Choice	Peer answers
Obtain a plasma level of olanzapine	68%
Raise the dose of olanzapine	16%
Switch to a different antipsychotic	13%
Add a mood-stabilizing anticonvulsant	3%

A – Correct. Obtaining antipsychotic plasma levels in patients who have had poor response despite a trial with an adequate dose/ duration of medication can be helpful in order to rule out poor adherence, identify rapid elimination, or confirm true treatment resistance. Although not all antipsychotics have well-established therapeutic plasma levels, olanzapine is among those agents that do.

B – Incorrect. Although raising the dose of olanzapine in a patient who has neither a response nor side effects could be attempted, plasma levels – not dose – are the best guide to the extent of patient medication exposure and are the best predictors of antipsychotic response. Thus, given that the olanzapine dose is at the top of the typically recommended range, one would ideally obtain plasma levels prior to any treatment adjustment.

C – Incorrect. Given that the patient has neither a response nor any side effects, it is reasonable that her medication exposure is subtherapeutic despite being dosed in the therapeutic range. Thus, it would make sense to obtain antipsychotic plasma levels prior to switching medications.

D – Incorrect. While an augmentation treatment strategy might help, it is important to first obtain antipsychotic plasma levels to determine whether the patient is actually treatment-resistant to the medication, or the dose needs to be adjusted to achieve a therapeutic response.

References

Stahl SM. *Essential psychopharmacology, the prescriber's guide*, seventh edition. New York, NY: Cambridge University Press; 2020.

Stahl SM. *Stahl's essential psychopharmacology*, fifth edition. New York, NY: Cambridge University Press; 2021. (Chapter 5)

QUESTION FIFTEEN

A 38-year-old man was diagnosed with schizophrenia 14 years ago, and over the course of his illness has taken several different antipsychotics, all with partial response and no severe side effects. He now presents with acute exacerbation of hallucinations and delusions. He recently had bowel resection due to a gastrointestinal disorder, and blood levels reveal that he is not absorbing his medications well. One option for this patient would be to prescribe heroic oral doses of his antipsychotic. Aside from this approach, which of the following antipsychotics have formulations that may be good long-term options for bypassing his problem with absorption?

A. Asenapine, paliperidone, risperidone

B. Paliperidone, risperidone, quetiapine

C. Risperidone, quetiapine, ziprasidone

D. Quetiapine, ziprasidone, asenapine

Psychosis and Its Treatment

Answer to Question Fifteen

The correct answer is A.

Choice	Peer answers
Asenapine, paliperidone, risperidone	70%
Paliperidone, risperidone, quetiapine	13%
Risperidone, quetiapine, ziprasidone	10%
Quetiapine, ziprasidone, asenapine	7%

A – Correct. For patients with difficulty absorbing medications, the best options in order to reach therapeutic blood levels would be to prescribe heroic oral doses or to use parenteral, sublingual, or suppository administration. Asenapine has a sublingual formulation and a transdermal patch, while several atypical antipsychotics are available as long-acting injectable (LAI) antipsychotics: risperidone microspheres (2-week formulation), paliperidone palmitate (4-week and 12-week formulations), olanzapine pamoate (4-week formulation), aripiprazole monohydrate (4-week formulation), and aripiprazole lauroxil (4-, 6-, and 8-week formulations). Additional antipsychotics with LAI formulations include fluphenazine, haloperidol, flupenthixol, pipothiazine, and zuclopenthixol. Clozapine, olanzapine, and risperidone have orally disintegrating tablets; however, these medications are not absorbed sublingually and must be swallowed in order to undergo absorption in the gut. Chlorpromazine has a suppository formulation, and other antipsychotics may also be able to be administered as suppositories.

B – Incorrect. Paliperidone and risperidone are both viable options, but quetiapine is only available as an oral tablet.

C – Incorrect. Risperidone is a viable option. However, quetiapine is only available as an oral tablet. Ziprasidone is available in an intramuscular formulation, which would bypass absorption issues, but it is for acute agitation and is not to be administered long term.

D – Incorrect. Asenapine is a viable option, but neither quetiapine nor ziprasidone would be (see above for explanation).

References

Maroney M. An update on the current treatment strategies and emerging agents for the management of schizophrenia. *Am J Manag Care* 2020;26(3 Suppl): S55–61.

Stahl SM. *Case studies: Stahl's essential psychopharmacology*. New York, NY: Cambridge University Press; 2011.

Stahl SM. *Essential psychopharmacology, the prescriber's guide*, seventh edition. New York, NY: Cambridge University Press; 2017.

Stahl SM. *Stahl's essential psychopharmacology*, fifth edition. New York, NY: Cambridge University Press; 2021. (Chapter 5)

Psychosis and Its Treatment

QUESTION SIXTEEN

A 28-year-old man was recently diagnosed with schizophrenia. He has a body mass index of 30, fasting triglycerides of 220 mg/dL, and fasting glucose of 114 mg/dL. Which of the following is least likely to worsen his metabolic profile?

A. Olanzapine

B. Quetiapine

C. Risperidone

D. Ziprasidone

Answer to Question Sixteen

The correct answer is D.

Choice	Peer answers
Olanzapine	11%
Quetiapine	6%
Risperidone	9%
Ziprasidone	74%

A – Incorrect. Olanzapine is one of the antipsychotics most associated with weight gain and metabolic risk and would not be a first-line option for patients who have a primary concern about metabolic issues. Clozapine also can cause problematic weight and metabolic side effects.

B – Incorrect. Quetiapine can lead to weight gain and increased triglyceride levels and may be a second-line option if a primary concern is metabolic issues.

C – Incorrect. Risperidone can lead to weight gain and increased triglyceride levels and may be a second-line option if a primary concern is metabolic issues. Paliperidone, which is the active metabolite of risperidone, can also lead to weight gain and metabolic changes. Iloperidone, asenapine, cariprazine, and brexpiprazole may also cause weight gain.

D – Correct. Ziprasidone in general seems to be weight neutral and has been shown to lower triglyceride levels. It is therefore a recommended choice for individuals for whom metabolic issues are a primary concern. Other newer antipsychotics that may be less likely to cause weight gain or metabolic side effects include aripiprazole (although data suggest that weight gain may occur more in children and adolescents), lurasidone, and lumateperone.

References

Stahl SM. *Essential psychopharmacology, the prescriber's guide*, seventh edition. New York, NY: Cambridge University Press; 2017.

Stahl SM. *Stahl's essential psychopharmacology*, fifth edition. New York, NY: Cambridge University Press; 2021. (Chapter 5)

QUESTION SEVENTEEN

A 37-year-old woman with schizophrenia has failed to respond to two sequential adequate trials of antipsychotic monotherapy (first olanzapine, then aripiprazole). Which of the following are evidence-based treatment strategies for a patient in this situation?

A. High dose of her current monotherapy (aripiprazole)

B. Augmentation of her current monotherapy with another atypical antipsychotic

C. Switch to clozapine

D. A and C

E. A, B, and C

Answer to Question Seventeen

The correct answer is C.

Choice	Peer answers
High dose of her current monotherapy (aripiprazole)	1%
Augmentation of her current monotherapy with another atypical antipsychotic	9%
Switch to clozapine	66%
A and C	10%
A, B, and C	15%

A – Incorrect. Controlled studies for high doses of antipsychotics are quite limited. In particular, the limited data that exist for aripiprazole suggest that it is not usually more effective at doses above the usual recommended range (i.e., 15–30 mg/day for psychosis). Before resorting to high-dose monotherapy, evidence-based strategies for treatment resistance should be exhausted, including the use of clozapine.

B – Incorrect. There is limited evidence to support the superior efficacy of combining antipsychotics vs. switching to clozapine or another monotherapy. Controlled studies are limited and review of the evidence that does exist (clinical trials and case reports) has not led to recommendations for antipsychotic polypharmacy in routine clinical practice.

C – Correct. After failure of two sequential adequate trials of antipsychotic monotherapy, the recommended and evidence-based treatment strategy is to switch to clozapine.

D and E – Incorrect.

References

Pandurangi AK, Dalkilic A. Polypharmacy with second-generation antipsychotics: a review of evidence. *J Psychiatr Pract* 2008;14:345.

Royal College of Psychiatrists. CR138. Consensus Statement on High-Dose Antipsychotic Medication. 2006. Available at: www.rcpsych.ac.uk/docs/default-source/members/faculties/rehabilitation-and-social-psychiatry/rehab-cr190.pdf?sfvrsn=d8397218_4.

Stahl SM. *Essential psychopharmacology, the prescriber's guide*, seventh edition. New York, NY: Cambridge University Press; 2020.

QUESTION EIGHTEEN

Carol is a 47-year-old patient with schizophrenia. She was taking a conventional antipsychotic but decided to stop taking it when she developed parkinsonian symptoms. Secondary to stopping her conventional antipsychotic, Carol's auditory hallucinations and paranoia returned, and she was rehospitalized. You recommend that she be started on an atypical antipsychotic. Which of the following has the lowest risk of drug-induced parkinsonism associated with it?

A. Asenapine

B. Iloperidone

C. Olanzapine

D. Paliperidone

Answer to Question Eighteen

The correct answer is B.

Choice	Peer answers
Asenapine	16%
Iloperidone	42%
Olanzapine	29%
Paliperidone	13%

As a class, atypical antipsychotics tend to have a decreased risk of movement disorders relative to conventional antipsychotics; however, the risk differs with each individual agent.

A, C, and D – Incorrect.

B – Correct. Of the agents listed here (asenapine, iloperidone, olanzapine, paliperidone), iloperidone has a relatively lower risk of drug-induced parkinsonism. Other agents with a relatively lower risk of drug-induced parkinsonism include clozapine, lumateperone, and quetiapine.

References

Roth BL. Ki determinations, receptor binding profiles, agonist and/or antagonist functional data, HERG data, MDR1 data, etc. as appropriate was generously provided by the National Institute of Mental Health's Psychoactive Drug Screening Program, Contract # HHSN-271–2008–00025-C (NIMH PDSP). The NIMH PDSP is directed by Bryan L. Roth, MD, PhD at the University of North Carolina at Chapel Hill and Project Officer Jamie Driscol at NIMH, Bethesda, MD, USA. For experimental details please refer to the PDSP website http://pdsp.med.unc.edu.

Santana N, Mengod G, Artigas F. Expression of alpha 1-adrenergic receptors in rat prefrontal cortex: cellular co-localization with 5-HT$_{2A}$ receptors. *Int J Neuropsychopharmacol* 2013;16(5):1139–51.

Stahl SM. *Stahl's essential psychopharmacology*, fifth edition. New York, NY: Cambridge University Press; 2021. (Chapter 5)

QUESTION NINETEEN

Ryan is a 26-year-old white male with treatment-resistant schizoaffective disorder, depressive type, and frequent suicidal ideation and behavior. After adequate but unsuccessful trials with several mood stabilizers and atypical antipsychotics (both as monotherapy and in various combinations), you are considering a trial of clozapine. Which of the following testing should you order prior to initiating clozapine?

A. White blood cell count (WBC)

B. Absolute neutrophil count (ANC)

C. A and B

D. Neither A nor B

Psychosis and Its Treatment

Answer to Question Nineteen

The correct answer is B.

Choice	Peer answers
White blood cell count (WBC)	2%
Absolute neutrophil count (ANC)	49%
A and B	49%
Neither A nor B	0%

A – Incorrect. Total WBC is no longer used when deciding whether to initiate or continue clozapine.

B – Correct. Before initiating clozapine treatment, it is necessary to obtain ANC. The lower ANC threshold for starting clozapine is at least 1500/μL in the general population and at least 1000/μL in individuals with benign ethnic neutropenia (BEN). BEN is a condition observed in certain ethnic groups (most commonly those of African descent, some Middle Eastern ethnic groups, and other non-Caucasian ethnic groups with darker skin). Patients with BEN have normal hematopoietic stem cell numbers and myeloid maturation, are healthy, do not suffer from repeated or severe infections, and are not at an increased risk for developing clozapine-induced neutropenia.

C – Incorrect. ANC, but not WBC, is required prior to initiating clozapine.

D – Incorrect. ANC is required prior to initiating clozapine.

References
Neuroscience Education Institute. Recommended ANC monitoring [pdf]. 2017.
Stahl SM. *Essential psychopharmacology, the prescriber's guide*, seventh edition. New York, NY: Cambridge University Press; 2020.

QUESTION TWENTY

A 38-year-old woman was diagnosed with schizophrenia approximately 2 years ago, and after multiple trials of atypical and typical antipsychotic medications she has been maintained on haloperidol for the last several months with good response. Two weeks ago, she began exhibiting mild motor symptoms of drug-induced parkinsonism. Which of the following would be the most appropriate adjunct medication for this patient?

A. Alpha 1 adrenergic agonist

B. Cholinesterase inhibitor

C. Histamine 1 antagonist

D. Muscarinic 1 antagonist

Answer to Question Twenty

The correct answer is D.

Choice	Peer answers
Alpha 1 adrenergic agonist	10%
Cholinesterase inhibitor	24%
Histamine 1 antagonist	11%
Muscarinic 1 antagonist	55%

Drug-induced parkinsonism is associated with a relative deficiency of dopamine and an excess of acetylcholine in the nigrostriatal pathway. Dopamine normally suppresses acetylcholine activity; thus, blockade of dopamine 2 receptors by antipsychotics enhances release of acetylcholine and can lead to the production of parkinsonian symptoms. Increasing availability of dopamine and/or decreasing acetylcholine would therefore be expected to relieve drug-induced parkinsonism.

A – Incorrect. Haloperidol is an antagonist at the alpha 1 adrenergic receptor and an agonist would therefore reverse its effects; however, alpha 1 stimulation may actually decrease striatal dopamine release and thus would not relieve parkinsonism.

B – Incorrect. A cholinesterase inhibitor would reduce metabolism of acetylcholine and cause a further increase, rather than decrease, in this neurotransmitter.

C – Incorrect. Similarly, the histamine system is not associated with development of, or relief from, drug-induced parkinsonism. Some antihistamines are muscarinic 1 antagonists but their histamine 1 antagonist properties do not regulate extrapyramidal side effects.

D – Correct. Antagonism of the muscarinic 1 receptor for acetylcholine would prevent it from binding there and thus reduce its effects, potentially relieving drug-induced parkinsonism.

References

Stahl SM. *Essential psychopharmacology, the prescriber's guide*, seventh edition. New York, NY: Cambridge University Press; 2017.

Stahl SM. *Stahl's essential psychopharmacology*, fifth edition. New York, NY: Cambridge University Press; 2021. (Chapter 5)

Psychosis and Its Treatment

QUESTION TWENTY-ONE

With long-acting injectable (LAI) antipsychotics, the time to steady state is a function of:

A. Elimination rate

B. Absorption rate

Answer to Question Twenty-One

The correct answer is B.

Choice	Peer answers
Elimination rate	25%
Absorption rate	75%

A – Incorrect. Typically, when an immediate-release medication is administered *orally*, it is absorbed rapidly. How long it takes to remove the medication from the body is therefore largely dependent on the rate of elimination. This also means that the time to steady state with repeated dosing is a function of elimination rate. However, with LAI antipsychotics, the rate of absorption is much slower than the rate of elimination, which leads to something called "flip-flop" kinetics. That is, because the medication cannot be eliminated until it is absorbed, the terminal slope is largely dependent on the absorption rate. In this case, the time to steady state is a function of *absorption* rate.

The long half-lives of LAI antipsychotics mean that, when converting from oral formulations, one must either adequately load the dose, if possible, or provide oral supplementation. A loading dose is the dose required to immediately achieve a plasma concentration that is equivalent to the steady-state concentration. The failure to adequately load the dose or provide oral supplementation can lead to subtherapeutic antipsychotic plasma levels for weeks or months.

B – Correct. Time to steady state for LAI antipsychotics is a function of absorption rate.

References

Meyer JM. Converting oral to long-acting injectable antipsychotics: a guide for the perplexed. *CNS Spectr* 2017;22(Suppl):17–27.

Spanarello S, La Ferla T. The pharmacokinetics of long-acting antipsychotic medications. *Curr Clin Pharmacol* 2014;9(3):310–17.

Psychosis and Its Treatment

QUESTION TWENTY-TWO

Reggie is a 30-year-old male patient with schizophrenia. He is currently taking iloperidone 24 mg/day as well as aripiprazole 15 mg/day but continues to experience visual hallucinations. To improve this patient's psychosis, it is likely necessary to further increase the blockade of dopamine D2 receptors. Which treatment strategy is likely the best course of action?

A. Increase iloperidone dose while keeping aripiprazole dose the same

B. Increase iloperidone and aripiprazole doses

C. Increase aripiprazole dose while keeping iloperidone dose the same

D. Maintain iloperidone dose and discontinue aripiprazole

Psychosis and Its Treatment

Answer to Question Twenty-Two

The correct answer is D.

Choice	Peer answers
Increase iloperidone dose while keeping aripiprazole dose the same	27%
Increase iloperidone and aripiprazole doses	2%
Increase aripiprazole dose while keeping iloperidone dose the same	29%
Maintain iloperidone dose and discontinue aripiprazole	42%

Aripiprazole is a D2 partial agonist and is also one of the most potent agents that bind to D2 receptors. Thus, when given concomitantly with a D2 antagonist, such as iloperidone, it can actually reduce the level of D2 blockade compared to D2 antagonist monotherapy, thus reducing the antipsychotic efficacy.

A – Incorrect. Increasing the dose of iloperidone while maintaining the aripiprazole dose would not likely lead to a relevant increase in D2 blockade (and corresponding improvement of psychotic symptoms), since aripiprazole has higher affinity for the D2 receptor.

B – Incorrect. Increasing doses of both iloperidone and aripiprazole would not likely lead to improvement of psychotic symptoms, since aripiprazole would continue to compete with iloperidone at the D2 receptor.

C – Incorrect. Increasing the dose of aripiprazole may actually decrease D2 blockade rather than increase it, since aripiprazole has higher affinity for the D2 receptor than iloperidone.

D – Correct. Because aripiprazole may be reducing the level of D2 blockade relative to iloperidone monotherapy, the best strategy for increasing D2 blockade (and correspondingly improving psychotic symptoms) may be to use monotherapy.

Reference
Stahl SM. *Stahl's essential psychopharmacology*, fifth edition. New York, NY: Cambridge University Press; 2021. (Chapter 5)

QUESTION TWENTY-THREE

Lumateperone has a unique mechanism of action that targets three neurotransmitter pathways through modulation of dopamine D1 and D2 receptors and glutamate (NMDA) receptor subunit epsilon-2, also known as N-methyl-D-aspartate receptor subtype 2B (GLuN2B), via downstream dopamine D1 receptors and through α-amino-3-hydroxy-5-methyl-4-isoxazolepropionic acid (AMPA) currents via the mTOR protein pathway. It is also a selective serotonin (5HT) 5HT2A receptor antagonist. Which component hypothetically may contribute to improved cognition?

A. Dopamine phosphoprotein D2 modulator (DPPM)

B. 5HT2A receptor antagonist

C. Glutamatergic phosphoprotein modulator

D. Serotonin reuptake inhibitor

Answer to Question Twenty-Three

The correct answer is C.

Choice	Peer answers
Dopamine phosphoprotein D2 modulator (DPPM)	14%
5HT2A receptor antagonist	22%
Glutamatergic phosphoprotein modulator	57%
Serotonin reuptake inhibitor	7%

A – Incorrect. Lumateperone acts as a D2 presynaptic partial agonist and a D2 postsynaptic antagonist selectively in the mesolimbic and mesocortical areas. This mechanism is not posited to be related to potential differential effects on cognition.

B – Incorrect. 5HT2A receptor antagonism is a property shared across the atypical antipsychotic class. This property enhances antipsychotic activity, reducing positive symptoms, while enhancing antidepressant activity. It may also be related to improved sleep quality, reduced anxiety, and reduced agitation. It is not posited to be related to improved cognition.

C – Correct. As a glutamatergic phosphoprotein modulator, lumateperone increases phosphorylation of mesolimbic GluN2B subunits of NMDA receptors resulting in indirect enhancement of glutamatergic NMDA function, along with NMDA and AMPA receptor enhancement via downstream D1 receptors. This may result in improved cognition as well as a reduction in positive and negative symptoms. It may also contribute to rapid-acting antidepressant activity.

D – Incorrect. Serotonin reuptake inhibition is not related to improved cognition.

References

Krogmann A, Peters L, von Hardenberg L et al. Keeping up with the therapeutic advances in schizophrenia: a review of novel and emerging pharmacological entities. *CNS Spectr* 2019;24(S1):38–69.

Maroney M. An update on the current treatment strategies and emerging agents for the management of schizophrenia. *Am J Manag Care* 2020;26(3 Suppl):S55–61.

Muly EC, Votaw JR, Ritchie J, Howell LL. Relationship between dose, drug levels, and D2 receptor occupancy for the atypical antipsychotics risperidone and paliperidone. *J Pharmacol Exp Ther* 2012;341(1):81–9.

Snyder GL, Vanover KE, Hongwen Z et al. Functional profile of a novel modulator of serotonin, dopamine, and glutamate neurotransmission. *Psychopharmacology (Berl)* 2015;232(3):605–21.

QUESTION TWENTY-FOUR

A 33-year-old man who was recently diagnosed with schizophrenia is taking 10 mg of sublingual asenapine twice a day. He reports a
marked reduction in positive symptoms, and no motor side effects.
Unfortunately, he also reports that he has noticed a numbness in his
mouth, a loss of taste, and there are blisters under his tongue. Which
treatment strategy is likely the best course of action?

A. Reduce the sublingual asenapine dose to 5 mg twice a day

B. Chew or swallow the medication in order to avoid the oral
   adverse effects he is experiencing

C. Switch to the FDA-approved asenapine transdermal patch

D. Only administer the sublingual asenapine dose once a day

Answer to Question Twenty-Four

The correct answer is C.

Choice	Peer answers
Reduce the sublingual asenapine dose to 5 mg twice a day	3%
Chew or swallow the medication in order to avoid the oral adverse effects he is experiencing	2%
Switch to the FDA-approved asenapine transdermal patch	93%
Only administer the sublingual asenapine dose once a day	3%

A – Incorrect. Reducing the dose may reduce the adverse oral side effects he is experiencing, but it may also reduce the alleviation of positive symptoms. The recommended therapeutic dose to alleviate positive symptoms of schizophrenia is 10 mg twice a day for a total of 20 mg per day.

B – Incorrect. Patients should be instructed to place the tablet under the tongue and allow it to dissolve completely, which will occur in seconds. The tablet should not be divided, crushed, chewed, or swallowed. Asenapine is not absorbed after swallowing (less than 2% bioavailable orally) and thus must be administered sublingually (35% bioavailable), as swallowing would render asenapine inactive. Patients may not eat or drink for 10 minutes following sublingual administration so that the drug in the oral cavity can be absorbed locally and not washed into the stomach (where it would not be absorbed).

C – Correct. The asenapine transdermal system is the only transdermal medication approved for schizophrenia. Transdermal delivery systems may have benefits over other formulations, such as the ability to visually confirm medication adherence and possible improved tolerability. Adverse oral events, such as the hypoesthesia and dysgeusia associated with the sublingual asenapine, could be avoided by utilizing the transdermal patch. Since this patient has benefited from the effects of asenapine, a non-oral formulation of asenapine, such as the transdermal patch, may be ideal to avoid the oral side effects he has been experiencing.

D – Incorrect. Once daily use seems theoretically possible because the half-life of asenapine is 13–39 hours, but this has not been extensively studied and may be limited by the need to expose the limited sublingual surface area to a limited amount of sublingual drug dosage.

References

Maroney M. An update on the current treatment strategies and emerging agents for the management of schizophrenia. *Am J Manag Care* 2020;26(3 Suppl): S55–61.

Stahl SM. *Essential psychopharmacology, the prescriber's guide*, seventh edition. New York, NY: Cambridge University Press; 2020.

CHAPTER PEER COMPARISON

For the Psychosis section, the correct answer was selected 63% of the time.

Psychosis and Its Treatment

8 SLEEP/WAKE DISORDERS AND THEIR TREATMENT

QUESTION ONE

Denise is a 32-year-old patient with shift work disorder who reports that she is having difficulty in her job as a pastry chef due to excessive sleepiness during her shift. Which of the following is a potential therapeutic mechanism to promote wakefulness?

A. Inhibit gamma-aminobutyric acid (GABA) activity

B. Inhibit histamine activity

C. Inhibit orexin activity

Answer to Question One

The correct answer is A.

Choice	Peer answers
Inhibit gamma-aminobutyric acid (GABA) activity	66%
Inhibit histamine activity	14%
Inhibit orexin activity	20%

The hypothalamus is a key control center for sleep and wake, and the specific circuitry that regulates sleep/wake is called the sleep/wake switch. The "off" setting, or sleep promoter, is localized within the ventrolateral preoptic nucleus (VLPO) of the hypothalamus, while "on" – the wake promoter – is localized within the tuberomammillary nucleus (TMN) of the hypothalamus. Two key neurotransmitters regulate the sleep/wake switch: histamine from the TMN and GABA from the VLPO.

A – Correct. When the VLPO is active and GABA is released to the TMN, the sleep promoter is on and the wake promoter is inhibited. Thus, inhibiting GABA activity can promote wakefulness.

B – Incorrect. When the TMN is active and histamine is released to the cortex and the VLPO, the wake promoter is on and the sleep promoter is inhibited. Thus, inhibiting histamine activity can promote sleep, not wakefulness.

C – Incorrect. The sleep/wake switch is also regulated by orexin neurons in the lateral hypothalamus, which stabilize wakefulness. Inhibition of orexin would therefore promote sleep, not wakefulness. In fact, a deficiency of orexin is an underlying cause of the extreme and sudden sleepiness seen in narcolepsy.

References
Stahl SM. *Stahl's essential psychopharmacology*, fifth edition. New York, NY: Cambridge University Press; 2021. (Chapter 10)

Stahl SM, **Morrissette DA**. *Stahl's illustrated sleep and wake disorders*. Cambridge, UK: Cambridge University Press; 2016.

QUESTION TWO

A 72-year-old man has been having difficulty sleeping for several weeks, including both difficulty falling asleep and frequent nighttime awakenings. Medical examination rules out an underlying condition contributing to insomnia, and he is not taking any medications that are associated with disrupted sleep. The patient is retired and spends the day caring for his grandchildren, including occasionally driving the older ones to school in the mid-morning. Which of the following would be the most appropriate treatment option for this patient?

A. Flurazepam

B. Temazepam

C. Zaleplon

D. Zolpidem CR

Answer to Question Two

The correct answer is D.

Choice	Peer answers
Flurazepam	1%
Temazepam	12%
Zaleplon	26%
Zolpidem CR	62%

For GABA-A medications, such as the benzodiazepines (e.g., flurazepam, temazepam) and Z-drugs (e.g., zaleplon, zolpidem CR), the critical threshold of receptor occupancy for onset of hypnotic effects is 25–30%. Both the onset to achieving the threshold and the duration of time above the sleep threshold are important for efficacy and for safety. The ideal hypnotic agent would have a duration above the threshold of approximately 8 hours.

A – Incorrect. Hypnotics with ultra-long half-lives (greater than 24 hours: for example, flurazepam and quazepam) can cause drug accumulation with chronic use. This can cause impairment that has been associated with increased risk of falls, particularly in the elderly.

B – Incorrect. For hypnotics with moderately long half-lives (15–30 hours: for example, estazolam and temazepam), receptor occupancies above the sleep threshold may not wear off until after the individual needs to awaken, potentially leading to "hangover" effects (sedation, memory problems). Other medications with sedating properties that have moderate half-lives include most tricyclic antidepressants, mirtazapine, and olanzapine. Given that this patient sometimes needs to drive in the morning, an agent with a moderate half-life may not be the best option for him.

C – Incorrect. For hypnotics with ultra-short half-lives (1–3 hours: zaleplon, triazolam, zolpidem, melatonin, ramelteon), receptor occupancies above the sleep threshold may not last long enough, causing loss of sleep maintenance, which is already a problem for this patient.

D – Correct. Hypnotics with half-lives that are short but not ultra-short (approximately 6 hours: zolpidem CR, eszopiclone, and perhaps low doses of trazodone or doxepin) may provide rapid onset of action and plasma levels above the minimally effective concentration only for the duration of a normal night's sleep. Thus, of the answer choices, zolpidem CR may best treat the patient's difficulties with sleep onset and maintenance while avoiding risks associated with agents with longer half-lives. The dose of zolpidem CR in elderly patients is 6.25 mg/night.

References

Stahl SM. *Stahl's essential psychopharmacology, the prescriber's guide*, seventh edition. New York, NY: Cambridge University Press; 2020.

Stahl SM. *Stahl's essential psychopharmacology*, fifth edition. New York, NY: Cambridge University Press; 2021. (Chapter 10)

Sleep/Wake Disorders and Their Treatment

QUESTION THREE

A 75-year-old man in good physical shape is having sleep problems. He wakes up at 4am and although he tries to stay awake in the evening to prevent this early rising, he usually falls asleep right after dinner, often before 7pm. Which of the following treatment options may be most beneficial for this patient?

A. Early morning melatonin

B. Evening melatonin

C. Late afternoon/evening light

D. A and C

E. A and B

F. B and C

Answer to Question Three

The correct answer is D.

Choice	Peer answers
Early morning melatonin	2%
Evening melatonin	4%
Late afternoon/evening light	16%
A and C	51%
A and B	1%
B and C	26%

The sleep/wake cycle is mediated by two opposing drives: homeostatic sleep drive and circadian wake drive. The circadian wake drive is a result of input (light, melatonin, activity) to the suprachiasmatic nucleus (SCN) of the hypothalamus, which stimulates the release of orexin to stabilize wakefulness. Circadian rhythm disorders occur when the internal circadian clock is out of sync with external cues that signal daytime and nighttime.

Patients with advanced sleep phase disorder become sleepy and thus go to bed earlier than desired and also wake up earlier than desired; this is a common problem for elderly individuals. These individuals have adequate total sleep time and quality of sleep. Patients with delayed sleep phase disorder are unable to fall asleep until the early morning hours and have difficulty waking until late morning/early afternoon. This is common during the teenage years; these individuals have adequate total sleep time and quality of sleep; however, the shifted sleep schedule can often interfere with activities of daily functioning.

A and C – Partially correct.

B, E, and F – Incorrect. Evening melatonin would not be appropriate for this elderly patient with advanced sleep phase disorder, because the patient is not having difficulty falling asleep in the evening. Rather, evening melatonin (and morning light) may benefit patients with *delayed* sleep phase disorder, potentially resetting the SCN so that the sleep/wake switch turns on earlier.

D – Correct. This patient is phase advanced. Advanced sleep phase disorder may be treated with early morning melatonin and evening light, which could help reset the SCN so that the sleep/wake switch stays off longer.

References

Edwards BA, O'Driscoll DM, Ali A et al. Aging and sleep: physiology and pathophysiology. *Semin Respir Crit Care Med* 2010;31(5):618–33.

Stahl SM. *Case studies: Stahl's essential psychopharmacology.* New York, NY: Cambridge University Press; 2011.

Sleep/Wake Disorders and Their Treatment

QUESTION FOUR

A 45-year-old woman was prescribed doxepin 10 mg/night for insomnia. She reports that it helped only a little, so she has been increasing the dose, up to 100 mg/night, as an attempt to increase the hypnotic effects (with some success). She also reports dizzy spells and constipation. Which property does doxepin exhibit in higher doses that could be the cause of these side effects?

A. Inhibiting reuptake of serotonin and norepinephrine

B. 5HT2A and 5HT2C antagonism

C. Alpha 1 adrenergic and muscarinic 1 antagonism

D. 5HT2A and 5HT2B antagonism

Answer to Question Four

The correct answer is C.

Choice	Peer answers
Inhibiting reuptake of serotonin and norepinephrine	6%
5HT2A and 5HT2C antagonism	6%
Alpha 1 adrenergic and muscarinic 1 antagonism	86%
5HT2A and 5HT2B antagonism	2%

A, B, and D – Incorrect. Higher doses of doxepin inhibit reuptake of serotonin and norepinephrine, but such effects are not likely to explain these side effects.

C – Correct. Low-dose doxepin is selective for histamine 1 receptors, which is why it can act as a hypnotic. It is likely that alpha 1 adrenergic and muscarinic 1 receptor antagonism seen with higher doses of doxepin would explain these side effects.

References
Stahl SM. Selective histamine H1 antagonism: novel hypnotic and pharmacologic actions challenge classical notions of antihistamines. *CNS Spectr* 2008;13(12):1027–38.

Stahl SM. *Stahl's essential psychopharmacology, the prescriber's guide*, seventh edition. New York, NY: Cambridge University Press; 2020.

Stahl SM. *Stahl's essential psychopharmacology*, fifth edition. New York, NY: Cambridge University Press; 2021. (Chapter 10)

QUESTION FIVE

Mary is a 33-year-old patient who complains of excessive sleepiness. She recently suffered injuries from a motor vehicle accident where she fell asleep at the wheel. Administration of the Multiple Sleep Latency Test (MSLT) revealed sleep latency of 5 minutes. Clinical evaluation revealed cerebrospinal fluid (CSF) hypocretin/orexin (Hcrt/Ox) levels in the low range (108 pg/mL), and several sleep-onset REM periods (SOREMPs) on the polysomnography. After ruling out medical and psychiatric causes of hypersomnia for this patient, your most likely diagnosis would be:

A. Narcolepsy with cataplexy

B. Narcolepsy without cataplexy

C. Idiopathic hypersomnia

D. Kleine–Levin syndrome

Answer to Question Five

The correct answer is A.

Choice	Peer answers
Narcolepsy with cataplexy	50%
Narcolepsy without cataplexy	40%
Idiopathic hypersomnia	6%
Kleine–Levin syndrome	3%

A – Correct. Narcolepsy is characterized by excessive daytime sleepiness, intrusion of sleep during wake times, and abnormal rapid eye movement (REM), including SOREMPs. Narcolepsy can occur with or without cataplexy (loss of muscle tone triggered by emotion). A CSF Hcrt/Ox level of < 110 pg/mL is diagnostic for narcolepsy. Even without cataplexy, patients with narcolepsy demonstrate more than two SOREMPs on the MSLT, as well as a short sleep latency (≤ 8 minutes). This patient had a very short sleep latency (5 minutes), and several SOREMPs, which suggests that she has narcolepsy.

In addition to its role in wakefulness and motivated behaviors, orexin is also involved in stabilizing motor movements, allowing normal movement in the day (when orexin levels are high) and facilitating inhibition of motor movements at night (when orexin levels are low). When orexin levels are low due to the degeneration of orexin neurons, this allows intrusion of motor inhibition and loss of muscle tone during wakefulness, a condition known as cataplexy. This patient had a Hcrt/Ox level of 108 pg/mL, which is considered in the low range, and is indicative of cataplexy.

B – Incorrect. The patient meets the criteria for both narcolepsy and cataplexy.

C – Incorrect. Patients with idiopathic hypersomnia have Hcrt/Ox levels in the normal range (200–700 pg/mL). Patients with idiopathic hypersomnia also have less than two SOREMPs, and this patient had several.

D – Incorrect. Kleine–Levin syndrome is the most common form of hypersomnia. This rare disorder mostly affects adolescent boys and is characterized by bouts of hypersomnolence coupled with cognitive and mood disturbances, compulsive eating, hypersexuality, and disinhibited behavior. This patient does not exhibit this profile or behavior. Additionally, patients with forms of recurrent hypersomnia demonstrate less than two SOREMPs and have normal levels of Hcrt/Ox.

References

Stahl SM. *Stahl's essential psychopharmacology*, fifth edition. New York, NY: Cambridge University Press; 2021. (Chapter 10)

Stahl SM, Morrissette DA. *Stahl's illustrated sleep and wake disorders.* Cambridge, UK: Cambridge University Press; 2016.

Sleep/Wake Disorders and Their Treatment

QUESTION SIX

Neurotransmitters fluctuate not only on a circadian (24-hour) basis, but also throughout the sleep cycle. _____ levels steadily increase during the first couple of hours of sleep, plateau, and then steadily decline before waking.

A. GABA/galanin

B. Hypocretin/orexin

C. Acetylcholine

D. Histamine

Answer to Question Six

The correct answer is A.

Choice	Peer answers
GABA/galanin	67%
Hypocretin/orexin	24%
Acetylcholine	3%
Histamine	5%

A – Correct. GABA and galanin levels steadily increase during the first couple of hours of sleep, plateau, and then steadily decline before waking.

B – Incorrect. Unlike GABA/galanin levels, hypocretin/orexin levels steadily decrease during the first couple of hours of sleep, plateau, and then steadily increase before waking.

C – Incorrect. Acetylcholine levels fluctuate throughout the sleep cycle, reaching their lowest levels during stage 4 sleep and peaking during REM sleep.

D – Incorrect. Histamine levels fluctuate throughout the sleep cycle, peaking during stage 2 sleep, and are at their lowest during REM sleep.

References
Stahl SM. *Stahl's essential psychopharmacology*, fifth edition. New York, NY: Cambridge University Press; 2021. (Chapter 10)

Stahl SM, Morrissette DA. *Stahl's illustrated sleep and wake disorders*. Cambridge, UK: Cambridge University Press; 2016.

QUESTION SEVEN

A clinician is planning to prescribe eszopiclone for a 34-year-old male patient with insomnia. What is the correct starting dose for this patient?

A. 0.5 mg/night

B. 1 mg/night

C. 2 mg/night

D. 3 mg/night

Answer to Question Seven

The correct answer is B.

Choice	Peer answers
0.5 mg/night	13%
1 mg/night	76%
2 mg/night	8%
3 mg/night	3%

A – Incorrect (0.5 mg/night).

B – Correct. In 2014, the US Food and Drug Administration (FDA) reduced the recommended starting dose of eszopiclone from 2 mg/night to 1 mg/night for both men and women. This is because, in some patients, eszopiclone blood levels may be high enough the next morning to cause impairment in activities that require alertness, including driving. In 2013, the FDA issued new dosing requirements for zolpidem due to the risk of next-morning impairment. However, the label change applied only to dosing in women (5 mg IR, 6.25 mg XR).

C – Incorrect (2 mg/night). Prior to the revised dosing requirements in 2014, the recommended dose range for eszopiclone was 2–3 mg/night; however, that is no longer the case.

D – Incorrect (3 mg/night). Prior to the revised dosing requirements in 2014, the recommended dose range for eszopiclone was 2–3 mg/night; however, that is no longer the case.

Reference

Stahl SM. *Stahl's essential psychopharmacology, the prescriber's guide*, seventh edition. New York, NY: Cambridge University Press; 2020.

QUESTION EIGHT

A 28-year-old woman with chronic insomnia is hoping to find an effective treatment but is reluctant to try anything that might cause dependence. Her clinician is considering prescribing lemborexant, which acts as an antagonist at orexin receptors. Specifically, what type of orexin antagonists may be effective for treating patients with sleep/wake disorders?

A. Single orexin receptor antagonists selective for orexin 1 receptors

B. Single orexin receptor antagonists selective for orexin 2 receptors

C. Dual orexin receptor antagonists that block both orexin 1 and 2 receptors

D. A and B

E. B and C

Answer to Question Eight

The correct answer is E.

Choice	Peer answers
Single orexin receptor antagonists selective for orexin 1 receptors	6%
Single orexin receptor antagonists selective for orexin 2 receptors	6%
Dual orexin receptor antagonists that block both orexin 1 and 2 receptors	39%
A and B	12%
B and C	37%

A – Incorrect. Orexin is released widely in the brain, interacting with all the arousal neurotransmitters to stabilize wakefulness and regulate attention. Orexin is also involved in other behaviors, including feeding, motivation, and reward. Its postsynaptic actions are mediated by two types of G-protein-coupled receptors: orexin 1 and orexin 2. Orexin 1 receptors are highly expressed in the locus coeruleus, where noradrenergic neurons originate, and are thought to play only a supplementary role in sleep/wake regulation. Consistent with this, preclinical trials with single orexin receptor antagonists for orexin 1 receptors have not demonstrated an effect on sleep.

B – Partially correct. Orexin 2 receptors are highly expressed in the tuberomammillary nucleus (TMN), where histaminergic neurons originate. It is believed that the effect of orexin on wakefulness is largely mediated by activation of the TMN histaminergic neurons that express orexin 2 receptors. Presumably, orexin 2 receptors therefore play a pivotal role in sleep/wake regulation. Consistent with this, there are promising preclinical results of single orexin receptor antagonists for orexin 2 receptors.

C – Partially correct. Dual orexin receptor antagonists have evidence of efficacy in the treatment of insomnia. Three such agents, lemborexant, daridorexant, and suvorexant, are approved to treat insomnia. Suvorexant has comparable affinity for orexin 1 and orexin 2 receptors, while lemborexant has higher affinity for orexin 2 receptors than for orexin 1 receptors.

D – Incorrect.

E – Correct (B and C).

Reference

Stahl SM. *Stahl's essential psychopharmacology*, fifth edition. New York, NY: Cambridge University Press; 2021. (Chapter 10)

QUESTION NINE

A 22-year-old college student stays up all night completing his thesis paper and then has to work the following day. While taking his break in the employee lounge he falls asleep in his chair. His fatigue and urge to sleep are hypothetically related to accumulation of which of the following neurotransmitters?

A. Adenosine

B. Histamine

C. Melatonin

D. Orexin

Answer to Question Nine

The correct answer is A.

Choice	Peer answers
Adenosine	45%
Histamine	13%
Melatonin	26%
Orexin	16%

A – Correct. The sleep/wake cycle is mediated by two opposing drives: homeostatic sleep drive and circadian wake drive. Homeostatic sleep drive is dependent on the accumulation of adenosine, which increases the longer one is awake and decreases with sleep. Accumulated adenosine leads to disinhibition of the ventrolateral preoptic nucleus and thus the release of GABA in the tuberomammillary nucleus to inhibit wakefulness. Antagonists at adenosine receptors, therefore, can promote wakefulness by preventing accumulated adenosine from binding to its receptors. Caffeine is the most notable example of an adenosine receptor antagonist.

B – Incorrect. Histamine promotes wakefulness, not sleepiness.

C – Incorrect. Endogenous melatonin is secreted by the pineal gland and mainly acts in the suprachiasmatic nucleus (SCN) to regulate circadian rhythms. When light enters through the eye it is translated via the retinohypothalamic tract to the SCN within the hypothalamus. The SCN, in turn, signals the pineal gland to turn *off* melatonin production. During darkness, with no inhibitory input from the SCN, the pineal gland turns *on* melatonin production. Melatonin, in turn, can act on the SCN to reset circadian rhythms.

D – Incorrect. Orexin stabilizes wakefulness; it does not promote sleepiness.

References

Stahl SM. *Stahl's essential psychopharmacology*, fifth edition. New York, NY: Cambridge University Press; 2021. (Chapter 10)

Stahl SM, Morrissette DA. *Stahl's illustrated sleep and wake disorders*. Cambridge, UK: Cambridge University Press; 2016.

QUESTION TEN

Rachel is an obese 35-year-old woman who works the night shift as an emergency medical responder. Recent evidence indicates that a disrupted sleep/wake cycle may increase one's risk for obesity, diabetes, and cardiovascular disease by:

A. Increasing levels of leptin

B. Increasing levels of ghrelin

C. Increasing levels of both leptin and ghrelin

D. Decreasing levels of both leptin and ghrelin

Answer to Question Ten

The correct answer is B.

Choice	Peer answers
Increasing levels of leptin	8%
Increasing levels of ghrelin	41%
Increasing levels of both leptin and ghrelin	45%
Decreasing levels of both leptin and ghrelin	6%

A – Incorrect. Leptin is an anorectic (appetite inhibiting) hormone. Increasing levels of leptin would therefore be expected to cause weight loss rather than obesity. Indeed, a disrupted sleep/wake cycle has been shown to *decrease* levels of leptin.

B – Correct. Ghrelin is an orexigenic (appetite stimulating) hormone. A disrupted sleep/wake cycle has been shown to increase levels of ghrelin; this increase in ghrelin is hypothesized to contribute to the increased risk of obesity, diabetes, and cardiovascular disease.

C and D – Incorrect. A disrupted sleep/wake cycle has been shown to decrease circulating levels of the anorectic (appetite inhibiting) hormone leptin and increase circulating levels of the orexigenic (appetite stimulating) hormone ghrelin.

References

Froy O. Metabolism and circadian rhythms – implications for obesity. *Endocr Rev* 2010;31(1):1–24.

Golombek DA, Casiraghi LP, Agostino PV et al. The times they are a-changing: effects of circadian desynchronization on physiology and disease. *J Physiol Paris* 2013;107:310–22.

Nixon JP, Mavanji V, Butterick TA et al. Sleep disorders, obesity, and aging: the role of orexin. *Aging Res Rev* 2015;20:63–73.

Orzel-Gryglewska J. Consequences of sleep deprivation. *Int J Occup Med Environ Health* 2010;23(1):95–114.

Stahl SM, Morrissette DA. *Stahl's illustrated sleep and wake disorders.* Cambridge, UK: Cambridge University Press; 2016.

QUESTION ELEVEN

A 12-year-old male patient has been brought to the clinic by his parents for evaluation. The patient typically sleeps for 10 or more hours a day (yet still exhibits excessive daytime sleepiness), eats excessive amounts of food, and demonstrates disinhibited behaviors including masturbation in public places. This patient most likely has:

A. Idiopathic hypersomnia

B. Narcolepsy without cataplexy

C. Kleine–Levin syndrome

Answer to Question Eleven

The correct answer is C.

Choice	Peer answers
Idiopathic hypersomnia	5%
Narcolepsy without cataplexy	3%
Kleine–Levin syndrome	92%

A – Incorrect. Idiopathic hypersomnia is characterized by either long or normal sleep duration accompanied by constant excessive daytime sleepiness, short sleep-onset latency, and complaints of non-refreshing sleep. Patients with idiopathic hypersomnia may also report sleep drunkenness and somnolence following sleep. The diagnosis of idiopathic hypersomnia includes excessive daytime sleepiness lasting at least 3 months; a sleep latency of under 8 minutes, as determined by the Multiple Sleep Latency Test (MSLT); and fewer than two sleep-onset REM periods (SOREMPs). Although some of the symptoms that this patient is experiencing, including excessive daytime sleepiness despite long sleep duration, are in line with idiopathic hypersomnia, the additional symptoms being exhibited by this patient (including disinhibited and compulsive behaviors) are suggestive of Kleine–Levin syndrome.

B – Incorrect. Narcolepsy is characterized by excessive daytime sleepiness, the intrusion of sleep during periods of wakefulness, and abnormal REM sleep, including periods of REM occurring at the onset of sleep (SOREMPs). Although some of the symptoms that this patient is experiencing, including excessive daytime sleepiness, are in line with narcolepsy, the additional symptoms being exhibited by this patient (including disinhibited and compulsive behaviors) are suggestive of Kleine–Levin syndrome.

C – Correct. Kleine–Levin syndrome is the most common form of recurrent hypersomnia. This rare disorder mostly affects adolescent boys and is characterized by bouts of hypersomnolence coupled with cognitive and mood disturbances, compulsive eating, hypersexuality, and disinhibited behavior.

References

Adenuga O, Attarian H. Treatment of disorders of hypersomnolence. *Curr Treat Options Neurol* 2014;16:302.

Dresler M, Spoormaker VI, Beitinger P et al. Neuroscience-driven discovery and development of sleep therapeutics. *Pharmacol Ther* 2014;141:300–34.

Larson-Prior LJ, Ju Y, Galvin JE. Cortical-subcortical interactions in hypersomnia disorders: mechanisms underlying cognitive and behavioral aspects of the sleep-wake cycle. *Frontiers Neurol* 2014;5(165):1–13.

Morgenthaler TI, Kapur VK, Brown T et al. Practice parameters for the treatment of narcolepsy and other hypersomnias of central origin. *Sleep* 2007;30(12):1705–11.

Stahl SM, Morrissette DA. *Stahl's illustrated sleep and wake disorders.* Cambridge, UK: Cambridge University Press; 2016.

Sleep/Wake Disorders and Their Treatment

QUESTION TWELVE

A 45-year-old patient has been unable to sleep more than 4 hours every night for the past 3 months. Chronic insomnia is believed to be due to:

A. Hypoarousal during the day

B. Hyperarousal at night

C. A and B

Answer to Question Twelve

The correct answer is B.

Choice	Peer answers
Hypoarousal during the day	1%
Hyperarousal at night	48%
A and B	51%

A – Incorrect. Insomnia is not due to hypoarousal during the day.

B – Correct. Insomnia is conceptualized as being related to hyper-arousal at night. Recent neuroimaging data suggest that insomnia is the result of an inability to switch off arousal-related circuits, rather than an inability to switch on sleep-related circuits. Some patients with insomnia experience hyperarousal during the day as well. To treat insomnia, one can administer medications that enhance the sleep drive, such as the GABAergic benzodiazepines or Z-drugs. Alternatively, one can administer medications that reduce arousal by inhibiting neurotransmission involved in wakefulness; notably, with antagonists at orexin, histamine, serotonin, or norepinephrine receptors.

C – Incorrect.

References
Stahl SM. *Stahl's essential psychopharmacology*, fifth edition. New York, NY: Cambridge University Press; 2021. (Chapter 10)

Stahl SM, Morrissette DA. *Stahl's illustrated sleep and wake disorders*. Cambridge, UK: Cambridge University Press; 2016.

Sleep/Wake Disorders and Their Treatment

QUESTION THIRTEEN

A 29-year-old male patient with shift work disorder exhibits excessive daytime sleepiness that is interfering with his ability to perform duties as a customer service agent. He is initiated on armodafinil with good therapeutic response. Modafinil and its R-enantiomer, armodafinil, are hypothesized to promote wakefulness and increase alertness by:

A. Decreasing dopamine

B. Decreasing hypocretin/orexin

C. Increasing histamine

D. All of the above

E. None of the above

Sleep/Wake Disorders and Their Treatment

Answer to Question Thirteen

The correct answer is C.

Choice	Peer answers
Decreasing dopamine	4%
Decreasing hypocretin/orexin	13%
Increasing histamine	49%
All of the above	16%
None of the above	18%

To promote wakefulness, one can administer medications that promote arousal by enhancing neurotransmission involved in wakefulness (most notably, by enhancing dopamine and histamine neurotransmission).

A – Incorrect. Modafinil and armodafinil bind with weak affinity to the dopamine transporter (DAT); however, their plasma levels are high and this compensates for the low binding. *Increased* synaptic dopamine following blockade of DAT leads to increased tonic firing and downstream effects on neurotransmitters involved in wakefulness, including histamine and orexin/hypocretin.

B – Incorrect. Orexin/hypocretin is a key component of the arousal system; thus, the hypothesized action of modafinil and armodafinil in increasing hypocretin/orexin may help promote alertness.

C – Correct. Modafinil and its R-enantiomer, armodafinil, are hypothesized to indirectly increase histamine, either by reducing GABAergic inhibition of histaminergic neurons or via actions at orexinergic neurons. The increase in histamine may contribute to both the wake-promoting effects of modafinil as well as the potential of modafinil to increase alertness.

D and E – Incorrect.

References

Bogan RK. Armodafinil in the treatment of excessive sleepiness. *Expert Opin Pharmacother* 2010;11(6):993–1002.

Stahl SM, Morrissette DA. *Stahl's illustrated sleep and wake disorders.* Cambridge, UK: Cambridge University Press; 2016.

QUESTION FOURTEEN

A 43-year-old man with narcolepsy is experiencing significant difficulties with daytime sleepiness and asks about potential pharmacological treatment. Which of the following would be a reasonable treatment option to address his daytime sleepiness?

A. Histamine 1 antagonist

B. Histamine 3 antagonist

C. Both A and B

D. Neither A nor B

Sleep/Wake Disorders and Their Treatment

Answer to Question Fourteen

The correct answer is B.

Choice	Peer answers
Histamine 1 antagonist	17%
Histamine 3 antagonist	36%
Both A and B	18%
Neither A nor B	29%

A – Incorrect. When histamine binds to postsynaptic histamine 1 receptors, it activates a G-protein-linked second messenger system that activates phosphatidyl inositol and the transcription factor cFOS. This results in wakefulness and normal alertness. Histamine 1 antagonists prevent activation of this second messenger and thus can cause sleepiness.

B – Correct. Histamine 3 receptors are presynaptic autoreceptors and function as gatekeepers for histamine. When H3 receptors are not bound by histamine, the molecular gate is open and allows histamine release. When histamine binds to the H3 receptor, the molecular gate closes and prevents histamine from being released. When an antagonist blocks the H3 receptor (e.g., pitolisant), this disinhibits, or turns on, the release of histamine, and can promote wakefulness.

C and D – Incorrect.

Reference

Stahl SM. *Stahl's essential psychopharmacology*, fifth edition. New York, NY: Cambridge University Press; 2021. (Chapter 10)

CHAPTER PEER COMPARISON

For the Sleep/Wake Disorders section, the correct answer was selected 58% of the time.

9   SUBSTANCE USE/IMPULSIVE-COMPULSIVE DISORDERS AND THEIR TREATMENT

QUESTION ONE

Your 16-year-old son is thrilled when he wins the 100-meter dash in an important high school competition. This "natural high" is most likely associated with inducing dopamine release in his mesolimbic pathway and in his:

A. Hypothalamus

B. Amygdala

C. Hippocampus

D. Cerebellum

E. Motor cortex

Answer to Question One

The correct answer is B.

Choice	Peer answers
Hypothalamus	12%
Amygdala	69%
Hippocampus	12%
Cerebellum	2%
Motor cortex	4%

A, C, D, and E – Incorrect. These brain regions are not known to be directly involved in the reactive reward system.

B – Correct. The brain can experience a "natural high" from activities such as athletic or intellectual accomplishments. This occurs when dopamine neurons release dopamine in the mesolimbic pathway, which is sometimes known as the "pleasure center" of the brain, and also in the amygdala, a critical component of the reactive reward system, which conditions reward responses in association with pleasurable activities.

References

Stahl SM. *Stahl's essential psychopharmacology*, fifth edition. New York, NY: Cambridge University Press; 2021.

Stahl SM, Grady MM. *Stahl's illustrated substance use and impulsive disorders.* New York, NY: Cambridge University Press; 2012. (Chapter 2)

QUESTION TWO

Impulsivity is hypothesized to be related to the _____, while compulsivity is hypothesized to be related to the _____.

A. Amygdala, ventral striatum

B. Ventral striatum, amygdala

C. Dorsal striatum, ventral striatum

D. Ventral striatum, dorsal striatum

Answer to Question Two

The correct answer is D.

Choice	Peer answers
Amygdala, ventral striatum	19%
Ventral striatum, amygdala	9%
Dorsal striatum, ventral striatum	20%
Ventral striatum, dorsal striatum	52%

Impulsivity and compulsivity can perhaps be best differentiated by how they both fail to control responses: impulsivity as the inability to stop initiating actions, and compulsivity as the inability to terminate ongoing actions. Impulsivity and compulsivity are hypothetically neurobiological drives that are "bottom-up," with impulsivity coming from the ventral striatum, compulsivity coming from the dorsal striatum, and different areas of the prefrontal cortex acting "top-down" to suppress these drives.

A – Incorrect. The amygdala is involved in reward conditioning and provides input to the striatum, but it is not directly associated with impulsivity. The dorsal striatum, not the ventral striatum, is associated with compulsivity.

B – Incorrect. Although the ventral striatum is linked to impulsivity, the amygdala is not directly linked to compulsivity.

C – Incorrect. Impulsivity is hypothesized to be related to the ventral striatum, while compulsivity is hypothesized to be related to the dorsal striatum.

D – Correct. Impulsivity is hypothesized to be related to the ventral striatum, while compulsivity is hypothesized to be related to the dorsal striatum.

Reference
Stahl SM. *Stahl's essential psychopharmacology*, fifth edition. New York, NY: Cambridge University Press; 2021.

QUESTION THREE

Mark, a 35-year-old cigarette smoker, would like to quit but is nervous because he typically craves a cigarette approximately every 2 hours. The craving and withdrawal are due to:

A. Desensitization of nicotinic receptors

B. Resensitization of nicotinic receptors

C. Desensitization of muscarinic receptors

D. Resensitization of muscarinic receptors

Answer to Question Three

The correct answer is B.

Choice	Peer answers
Desensitization of nicotinic receptors	27%
Resensitization of nicotinic receptors	65%
Desensitization of muscarinic receptors	3%
Resensitization of muscarinic receptors	5%

A – Incorrect. Cigarette smoking desensitizes all nicotinic alpha 4 beta 2 receptors and gets the maximum dopamine release. Receptors become desensitized so that they cannot function temporarily, and thus cannot react to either acetylcholine or nicotine. Putting nicotinic receptors out of business by desensitizing them causes neurons to attempt to overcome this lack of functioning receptors by upregulating the number of receptors.

B – Correct. During cigarette smoking cessation, resensitized nicotinic receptors no longer receiving nicotine are craving due to an absence of dopamine release in the nucleus accumbens. Craving seems to be initiated at the first sign of nicotinic receptor resensitization. When the receptors resensitize to their resting state, this initiates craving and withdrawal due to the lack of release of further dopamine.

C and D – Incorrect. Cigarette smoking does not have an effect on muscarinic receptors.

References

Narahashi T, Fenster CP, Quick MW et al. Symposium overview: mechanism of action of nicotine on neuronal acetylcholine receptors, from molecule to behavior. *Toxicol Sci* 2000;57(2):193–202.

Stahl SM. *Stahl's essential psychopharmacology*, fifth edition. New York, NY: Cambridge University Press; 2021.

QUESTION FOUR

A 56-year-old man presents to a new primary care provider for a routine physical exam. During the exam, he is asked some basic screening questions about alcohol use. The patient states that he drinks one mixed drink (containing a single 1-ounce shot) each night. How would you assess this patient's drinking behavior?

A. Low-risk drinking

B. At-risk drinking

C. Alcohol use disorder

Answer to Question Four

The correct answer is A.

Choice	Peer answers
Low-risk drinking	67%
At-risk drinking	30%
Alcohol use disorder	3%

Moderate alcohol consumption is defined as up to two drinks per day for men and up to one drink per day for women. Heavy alcohol use is defined as more than four drinks on any day for men or more than three drinks for women.

For men under the age of 65, the recommended drinking limits are no more than 4 drinks in one day and no more than 14 drinks in one week. For men aged 65 and older and for women, the recommended drinking limits are no more than three drinks per day and no more than seven drinks per week. Amounts in excess of these would be considered heavy or at-risk drinking but may not necessarily constitute an alcohol use disorder.

A – Correct. This patient consumes seven drinks per week (one drink per night). Therefore, he would be considered to have low-risk drinking behavior.

B and C – Incorrect. Based on the recommended drinking limits, this patient's drinking behavior does not indicate at-risk drinking or an alcohol use disorder.

References
National Institute on Alcohol Abuse and Addiction (NIAAA). Available at: www.niaaa.nih.gov.

Stahl SM, Grady MM. *Stahl's illustrated substance use and impulsive disorders.* New York, NY: Cambridge University Press; 2012. (Chapter 3)

QUESTION FIVE

Lisa, who is 13, has been staying up later than usual, complaining that she can't sleep. Sometimes during the day she locks herself in her room for hours, only coming out to use the bathroom. Recently, her mother discovered boxes of hidden cereal, chips, and cookies in her closet. Her mother suspects that Lisa has an eating disorder, but she is not sure if Lisa is vomiting or not, and her weight appears to be normal. Upon psychiatric evaluation, Lisa has negative affect, functional impairment, elevated thin-ideal internalization, and body dissatisfaction. She says she is dieting, but that she is not fasting. Which eating disorder is she at high risk for?

A. Anorexia nervosa

B. Bulimia nervosa

C. Binge eating disorder

Answer to Question Five

The correct answer is C.

Choice	Peer answers
Anorexia nervosa	7%
Bulimia nervosa	36%
Binge eating disorder	57%

A – Incorrect. Specific predictive risk factors for anorexia nervosa (AN) include negative affect, functional impairment, and low body mass index (BMI). However, youth who are inherently lean, rather than purposely pursuing the thin ideal, are at risk for AN, thus dieting would not be a specific risk factor for AN. Lisa does not have a low BMI, suggesting that she is not at risk for AN.

B – Incorrect. Specific predictive risk factors for bulimia nervosa include: thin-ideal internalization, positive thinness expectancy, denial of thin-ideal costs, body dissatisfaction, dieting, negative affect, overeating, fasting, functional impairment, and mental health care. While Lisa suffers from negative affect, overeating, thin-ideal internalization, body dissatisfaction, and functional impairment, she is not fasting.

C – Correct. Specific predictive risk factors for binge eating disorder (BED) include: elevated thin-ideal internalization, body dissatisfaction, functional impairment, dieting, overeating, negative affect, and mental health care. While negative affect and functional impairment are risk factors for all eating disorders, since Lisa is overeating and hiding her eating habits, while openly dieting, she is at high risk for the development of BED.

References

Stahl SM, Grady MM. *Stahl's illustrated substance use and impulsive disorders.* New York, NY: Cambridge University Press; 2012. (Chapter 3)

Stice E, Marti CN, Durant S. Risk factors that predict future onset of each DSM-5 eating disorder. Predictive specificity in high-risk adolescent females. *J Abnorm Psychol* 2017;126(1):38–51.

QUESTION SIX

A 28-year-old painter presents with a severe drinking problem, and you affirm the need for pharmacotherapy. When you suggest naltrexone, he asks how this will help. Which might you use as part of your explanation?

A. Naltrexone blocks mu-opioid receptors to reduce the euphoria you might normally experience with heavy drinking

B. Naltrexone blocks metabotropic glutamate receptors (mGluR) to reduce the euphoria you might normally experience with heavy drinking

C. Naltrexone stimulates mu-opioid receptors to reduce the euphoria you might normally experience with heavy drinking

D. Naltrexone stimulates mGluR receptors to reduce the euphoria you might normally experience with heavy drinking

Answer to Question Six

The correct answer is A.

Choice	Peer answers
Naltrexone blocks mu-opioid receptors to reduce the euphoria you might normally experience with heavy drinking	89%
Naltrexone blocks metabotropic glutamate receptors (mGluR) to reduce the euphoria you might normally experience with heavy drinking	7%
Naltrexone stimulates mu-opioid receptors to reduce the euphoria you might normally experience with heavy drinking	4%
Naltrexone stimulates mGluR receptors to reduce the euphoria you might normally experience with heavy drinking	1%

A – Correct. Blocking mu-opioid receptors might reduce the desire to engage in heavy drinking activity, as doing so will be associated with reduced reward.

B and D – Incorrect. Naltrexone is a mu-opioid antagonist. Mu-opioid receptors theoretically contribute to the "high" or euphoria experienced with heavy drinking, similar to their function in opiate abuse.

C – Incorrect. Blocking mu-opioid receptors, not stimulating them, is the likely mechanism of naltrexone's efficacy.

References
Stahl SM. *Stahl's essential psychopharmacology*, fifth edition. New York, NY: Cambridge University Press; 2021.

Stahl SM, Grady MM. *Stahl's illustrated substance use and impulsive disorders*. New York, NY: Cambridge University Press; 2012. (Chapter 3).

QUESTION SEVEN

Sarah is a 24-year-old woman seeking treatment for opioid addiction. To manage withdrawal, she is prescribed buprenorphine. The addition of clonidine also functions to reduce the intensity of withdrawal via what action?

A. Inhibition of norepinephrine reuptake

B. Inhibition of dopamine reuptake

C. Alpha 2A agonism

D. Alpha 2A antagonism

Answer to Question Seven

The correct answer is C.

Choice	Peer answers
Inhibition of norepinephrine reuptake	3%
Inhibition of dopamine reuptake	4%
Alpha 2A agonism	61%
Alpha 2A antagonism	32%

A, B, and D – Incorrect.

C – Correct. The intensity and duration of withdrawal from most drugs, including opioids, are linked to drug half-life, with short half-life full agonists such as morphine or heroin producing much more intense and short-lasting withdrawal symptoms than either long-acting methadone, which has a less intense but much longer duration withdrawal, or buprenorphine, whose withdrawal is both less intense and shorter. The intensity but not the duration of withdrawal of both methadone and buprenorphine can be reduced by the addition of an alpha 2A agonist such as clonidine or lofexidine. These agents can reduce signs of autonomic hyperactivity during withdrawal and aid in the detoxification process.

References

Gowing L, Farrell M, Ali R, White JM. Alpha$_2$-adrenergic agonists for the management of opioid withdrawal. *Cochrane Database Syst Rev* 2016;(5):CD002024.

Hooten WM. Opioid management: initiating, monitoring, and tapering. *Phys Med Rehabil Clin N Am* 2020;31(2):265–77.

Stahl SM. *Stahl's essential psychopharmacology*, fifth edition. New York, NY: Cambridge University Press; 2021.

QUESTION EIGHT

A 39-year-old accountant you have been seeing for several years has recently disclosed her 10-year prescription opiate addiction to you. While she is quite functional, she continues to seek opiates in order to avoid withdrawal effects. Which of the following is true about her potential for recovery?

A. Opioid receptors can readapt to normal but need a reduction in the amount of opiate exposure over time in order to do so

B. Opioid receptors cannot readapt to normal after severe addiction but can reorganize to nearly full functionality with the aid of permanent pharmacotherapy

Answer to Question Eight

The correct answer is A.

Choice	Peer answers
Opioid receptors can readapt to normal but need a reduction in the amount of opiate exposure over time in order to do so	85%
Opioid receptors cannot readapt to normal after severe addiction but can reorganize to nearly full functionality with the aid of permanent pharmacotherapy	15%

A – Correct. The brain's elasticity allows for opioid receptors to readapt to normal after some time of abstinence from drug intake. This may be difficult to tolerate, so reinstituting another opioid, such as methadone, or a partial mu-opioid agonist, such as buprenorphine (in combination with naloxone), may assist the detoxification process.

B – Incorrect.

References

Hooten WM. Opioid management: initiating, monitoring, and tapering. *Phys Med Rehabil Clin N Am* 2020;31(2):265–77.

Stahl SM. *Stahl's essential psychopharmacology*, fifth edition. New York, NY: Cambridge University Press; 2021.

Stahl SM, Grady MM. *Stahl's illustrated substance use and impulsive disorders.* New York, NY: Cambridge University Press; 2012. (Chapter 4)

QUESTION NINE

Mary is a 33-year-old woman with alcohol use disorder. She consumes several drinks a day nearly every day of the week and has recently had her two children removed from her care. She is motivated to attempt to stop drinking in order to get her children back. She previously attempted to quit cold turkey on her own, and ended up in the emergency room with severe withdrawal symptoms. Considering these factors, would she be a good candidate for reduced-risk drinking as a goal?

A. Yes

B. No

Answer to Question Nine

The correct answer is B.

Choice	Peer answers
Yes	37%
No	63%

A – Incorrect. Because this patient has a history of severe alcohol withdrawal symptoms, she would not be a good candidate for reduced-risk drinking as a goal. In addition, if she does not stop drinking it is less likely that she will be able to have the children returned to her care.

B – Correct. Reduced-risk drinking as a goal is controversial. However, some patients will not agree to abstinence as a goal. For these patients, it can still be beneficial to work with them to reduce their drinking. Reduced-risk drinking may be a better goal for patients with less severe problem drinking, including at-risk drinkers. The strategy for achieving reduced-risk drinking for patients with alcohol use disorder involves agreeing on a plan. Give patients a choice in the goal if possible – this allows them to take part in decisions affecting their lives and also gives them more responsibility in the outcome. Some sample guidelines for reduced-risk drinking include the "three As": avoid having more than one drink in one hour, avoid drinking patterns (same people, same places, same time of day), and avoid drinking to deal with problems.

Contraindications for reduced-risk drinking (as opposed to abstinence) include: existing conditions that would be exacerbated by alcohol, use of disulfiram or other agents contraindicated with alcohol, history of failed attempts with reduced-risk drinking, pregnancy or breastfeeding, and a history of severe alcohol withdrawal symptoms. For patients who should pursue abstinence but refuse, one may try to have them agree to a trial period of abstinence and a trial period of reduced-risk drinking; it can be beneficial to use a written contract.

References

Ambrogne JA. Reduced-risk drinking as a treatment goal: what clinicians need to know. *J Subst Abuse Treat* 2002;22(1):45–53.

Stahl SM. *Stahl's essential psychopharmacology*, fifth edition. New York, NY: Cambridge University Press; 2021.

Stahl SM, Grady MM. *Stahl's illustrated substance use and impulsive disorders*. New York, NY: Cambridge University Press; 2012. (Chapter 3)

QUESTION TEN

Clara is at a party with some friends and decides to try "Molly." She was told that "Molly" is the pure form of ecstasy (3,4-methylene-dioxymethamphetamine [MDMA]), lacking many of the harmful additives that can be found in ecstasy. Upon taking the pill, Clara notices that while she is in a state of excited delirium she has a nosebleed, sweats profusely, and feels nauseated. She is disoriented and wonders why she is feeling so horrible after taking the pure form of the drug. Her symptoms are most likely attributed to:

A. A synthetic cathinone, such as methylone

B. Caffeine

C. Methamphetamine

Answer to Question Ten

The correct answer is A.

Choice	Peer answers
A synthetic cathinone, such as methylone	71%
Caffeine	1%
Methamphetamine	28%

A – Correct. While "Molly" is the pure crystal powder form of MDMA, and lacks harmful additives commonly found in MDMA, such as caffeine and methamphetamine, the compounds are replaced by dangerous synthetic cathinones, such as methylone. Synthetic cathinones can cause nosebleeds, paranoia, hallucinations, nausea, sweating, panic attacks, and even death.

B, C – Incorrect.

References

Baumann MH. Awash in a sea of "bath salts": implications for biomedical research and public health. *Addiction* 2014;109(10):1577–9.

Saha K, Li Y, Holy M et al. The synthetic cathinones, butylone and pentylone, are stimulants that act as dopamine transporter blockers but 5-HT transporter substrates. *Psychopharmacology (Berl)* 2019;236(3): 953–62.

QUESTION ELEVEN

Peter is a 17-year-old student who has been using spice (synthetic cannabinoid) over the past year. Synthetic cannabinoids such as spice may be associated with an increased risk of psychosis compared to natural marijuana because they:

A. Do not contain cannabidiol

B. Are full rather than partial agonists

C. A and B

D. Neither A nor B

Answer to Question Eleven

The correct answer is C.

Choice	Peer answers
Do not contain cannabidiol	6%
Are full rather than partial agonists	23%
A and B	62%
Neither A nor B	10%

A – Partially correct. Spice use may cause recurrence or exacerbation of preexisting psychotic symptoms, with studies suggesting a possible three times increased risk of subsequent psychosis. One factor that may explain why this is seen with spice but not generally with natural marijuana is that natural marijuana contains cannabidiol, which is thought to have antipsychotic properties. In contrast, synthetic cannabinoids do not contain cannabidiol.

B – Partially correct. Unlike natural marijuana, which is a partial agonist at the cannabinoid 1 (CB-1) receptor, synthetic cannabinoids are full agonists at CB-1. Therefore, they can potentially lead to excessive stimulation of the receptor. In addition, synthetic cannabinoids bind to the CB-1 receptor with 800 times greater affinity than natural marijuana.

C – Correct. Both A and B are correct.

D – Incorrect.

References

Loeffler G, Hurst D, Penn A, Yung K. Spice, bath salts, and the U.S. military: the emergence of synthetic cannabinoid receptor agonists and cathinones in the U.S. Armed Forces. *Mil Med* 2012;177(9):1041–8.

Seely KA, Lapoint J, Moran JH, Fattore L. Spice drugs are more than harmless herbal blends: a review of the pharmacology and toxicology of synthetic cannabinoids. *Prog Neuropsychopharmacol Biol Psychiatry* 2012;39(2):234–43.

Woo TM, Hanley JR. "How high do they look?": identification and treatment of common ingestions in adolescents. *J Pediatr Health Care* 2013;27:135–44.

QUESTION TWELVE

Eddie is a 43-year-old man who has a 22-year-old daughter with a history of cocaine addiction. He recently heard about a novel cocaine vaccine that is being studied and would like to know more about it. In describing the cocaine vaccine, you explain that a cocaine-induced "high" is experienced when:

A. At least 47% of dopamine transporters are occupied by cocaine

B. At least 97% of norepinephrine transporters are occupied by cocaine

C. Both of the above

Answer to Question Twelve

The correct answer is A.

Choice	Peer answers
At least 47% of dopamine transporters are occupied by cocaine	55%
At least 97% of norepinephrine transporters are occupied by cocaine	5%
Both of the above	40%

A – Correct. Studies have shown that the "high" associated with cocaine occurs when at least 47% of dopamine transporters in the brain are occupied by cocaine. When the cocaine vaccine is administered, it causes the production of antibodies that then bind to the vaccine. The antibodies produced in response to the vaccine do not cross into the brain; thus, antibody-bound cocaine remains in the periphery and may therefore reduce the percentage of cocaine-occupied dopamine transporters below the 47% threshold needed to induce a high. One potential advantage of the vaccine is that it prevents cocaine from entering the brain without affecting normal dopamine neurotransmission.

B – Incorrect. Although cocaine does bind to the norepinephrine transporter, it is the effects at the dopamine transporter that are primarily responsible for the induced high.

C – Incorrect.

References

Garinot M, Piras-Douce F, Probeck P et al. A potent novel vaccine adjuvant based on straight polyacrylate. *Int J Pharm X* 2020;2:100054.

Kimishima A, Olson ME, Janda KD. Investigations into the efficacy of multi-component cocaine vaccines. *Bioorg Med Chem Lett* 2018;28(16):2779–83.

Maoz A, Hicks MJ, Vallabhjosula S et al. Adenovirus capsid-based anti-cocaine vaccine prevents cocaine from binding to the nonhuman primate CNS dopamine transporter. *Neuropsychopharmacology* 2013;38:2170–8.

QUESTION THIRTEEN

A 26-year-old woman develops a dependence on opioids after taking them during her recovery from knee surgery. She attempts to stop using them on her own, but when she does stop or decreases her dose, she experiences nausea, muscle aches, sweating, diarrhea, insomnia, and depression. She and her practitioner decide that buprenorphine would be an appropriate treatment strategy. Which of the following is true?

A. The patient should have the buprenorphine implant Probuphine inserted immediately

B. The patient should initiate oral buprenorphine while down-titrating her current opioid

C. The patient should be in a mild withdrawal state prior to initiating buprenorphine

D. The patient should complete withdrawal before beginning buprenorphine treatment

Answer to Question Thirteen

The correct answer is C.

Choice	Peer answers
The patient should have the buprenorphine implant Probuphine inserted immediately	1%
The patient should initiate oral buprenorphine while down-titrating her current opioid	18%
The patient should be in a mild withdrawal state prior to initiating buprenorphine	73%
The patient should complete withdrawal before beginning buprenorphine treatment	8%

A – Incorrect. The implant Probuphine contains buprenorphine, a partial opioid agonist. Probuphine is indicated for the maintenance treatment of opioid dependence in patients who have achieved and sustained prolonged clinical stability on low to moderate doses of a transmucosal buprenorphine-containing product (i.e., doses of no more than 8 mg/day of a sublingual tablet). Probuphine is not appropriate for new entrants to treatment and patients who have not achieved and sustained prolonged clinical stability, while being maintained on buprenorphine sublingual 8 mg/day.

B – Incorrect. Buprenorphine is a partial opioid agonist. It has stronger affinity for the mu-opioid receptor than other opioids, and thus causes immediate withdrawal if not administered when the patient is already in withdrawal.

C – Correct. Buprenorphine is a partial opioid agonist. It has stronger affinity for the mu-opioid receptor than other opioids, and thus causes immediate withdrawal if not administered when the patient is already in withdrawal. If the patient is already experiencing withdrawal, however, it will relieve those symptoms. Buprenorphine is commonly combined with naloxone in order to reduce its diversion and intravenous abuse.

D – Incorrect.

References

Chavoustie S, Frost M, Snyder O et al. Buprenorphine implants in medical treatment of opioid addiction. *Expert Rev Clin Pharmacol* 2017;10(8):799–807.

Dodrill CL, Helmer DA, Kosten TR. Prescription pain medication dependence. *Am J Psychiatry* 2011;168(5):466–71.

Hooten WM. Opioid management: initiating, monitoring, and tapering. *Phys Med Rehabil Clin N Am* 2020;31(2):265–77.

Stahl SM, Grady MM. *Stahl's illustrated substance use and impulsive disorders.* New York, NY: Cambridge University Press; 2012. (Chapter 4)

QUESTION FOURTEEN

A 23-year-old woman has recently been diagnosed with binge eating disorder. Since the age of 16 she has had episodes where she eats far beyond the point of hunger, typically at night and when she is alone. The patient feels very guilty and disgusted with herself about her eating habits; this is reinforced by her family members, who tell her that she is just weak and should have more self-control. Is there evidence to support the idea that individuals can develop an addiction to food?

A. Yes

B. No

Answer to Question Fourteen

The correct answer is A.

Choice	Peer answers
Yes	97%
No	3%

A – Correct. Food has powerful reinforcing effects. The neurobiological basis of eating and appetite is linked not just to the hypothalamus, but also to the connections that hypothalamic circuits make to reward pathways. Following food deprivation, any food will activate reward pathways. However, palatable (i.e., high-fat, high-sugar) foods activate reward pathways more reliably and more potently than do unpalatable foods. Even without food deprivation, highly palatable foods will activate the release of endocannabinoids and ghrelin; this is not true of unpalatable foods.

There is also evidence that the neurobiological changes associated with the progression to compulsive drug use may similarly occur in individuals with compulsive eating behaviors. When exposed to food cues, obese individuals exhibit increased activation, compared to lean individuals, in regions that process palatability. In contrast, obese individuals exhibit decreased activation of reward circuits during actual food consumption. This is analogous to cravings and tolerance in patients with substance use disorders.

Of course, not everyone who is obese has an eating compulsion, since obesity is also related to genetics and to lifestyle factors such as exercise, caloric intake, and the specific content of consumed foods. In fact, studies of brain activation in response to images of food can differentiate between individuals with binge eating disorder and overweight controls; in particular, differences in activation have been noted in the right ventral striatum.

B – Incorrect.

References

Keel PK, Bodell LP, Forney KJ, Appelbaum J, Williams D. Examining weight suppression as a transdiagnostic factor influencing illness trajectory in bulimic eating disorders. *Physiol Behav* 2019;208:112565.

Livovsky DM, Pribic T, Azpiroz F. Food, eating, and the gastrointestinal tract. *Nutrients* 2020;12(4):986.

Lutter M, Nestler EJ. Homeostatic and hedonic signals interact in the regulation of food intake. *J Nutr* 2009;139(3):629–32.

Monteleone P, Piscitelli F, Scognamiglio P et al. Hedonic eating is associated with increased peripheral levels of ghrelin and the endocannabinoid 2-arachidonoyl-glycerol in healthy humans: a pilot study. *J Clin Endocrinol Metab* 2012;97:E917–24.

Weygandt M, Schaefer A, Schienle A, Haynes JD. Diagnosing different binge-eating disorders based on reward-related brain activation patterns. *Hum Brain Mapp* 2012;33:2135–46.

QUESTION FIFTEEN

Evan is a 27-year-old male suffering from posttraumatic stress disorder. He is undergoing 3,4-methylenedioxymethamphetamine (MDMA ["ecstasy"])-assisted psychotherapy to induce an empathic and safe psychological state to explore his painful traumatic memories in the presence of his therapist. MDMA is able to induce this psychological state primarily through which action?

A. Serotonin 1A partial agonism

B. Serotonin 2A agonism

C. Competitive inhibition of the dopamine transporter

D. Competitive inhibition of the serotonin transporter

Answer to Question Fifteen

The correct answer is D.

Choice	Peer answers
Serotonin 1A partial agonism	9%
Serotonin 2A agonism	32%
Competitive inhibition of the dopamine transporter	26%
Competitive inhibition of the serotonin transporter	33%

A – Incorrect. MDMA does not target serotonin 1A partial agonism.

B – Incorrect. MDMA does not target serotonin 2A agonism.

C – Incorrect. MDMA does not target competitive inhibition of the dopamine transporter.

D – Correct. MDMA targets the serotonin transporter as a competitive inhibitor and pseudosubstrate, binding at the same site where serotonin binds to this transporter, thus inhibiting serotonin reuptake. Once there in sufficient quantities, MDMA is also a competitive inhibitor of the vesicular transporter (VMAT2) for serotonin. MDMA displaces serotonin from the synaptic vesicles, causing serotonin release from synaptic vesicles into the cytoplasm pre-synaptically. Once in the synapse, the serotonin can play upon any serotonin receptors that are there, but the evidence suggests that this is mostly upon 5HT2A receptors, just like the hallucinogen.

References

Meyer JS. 3,4-methylenedioxymethamphetamine (MDMA): current perspectives. *Subst Abuse Rehabil* 2013;4:83–99.

Stahl SM, Grady MM. *Stahl's illustrated substance use and impulsive disorders.* New York, NY: Cambridge University Press; 2012. (Chapter 4)

QUESTION SIXTEEN

A 73-year-old woman, Laura, has had a history of alcohol abuse. When people age, their sensitivity to alcohol increases as their tolerance decreases, and alcohol takes longer to be metabolized. Many prescribed medications increase the negative effects of alcohol. Laura was recently prescribed desipramine, a tricyclic antidepressant. What are the adverse effects that Laura should be aware of in combining the prescription medication with alcohol, particularly in the first week of treatment?

A. Severe hepatotoxicity with therapeutic doses

B. Increased anticoagulant effects

C. Combined central nervous system (CNS) depression decreases psychomotor performance

D. Masked signs of delirium tremens

Answer to Question Sixteen

The correct answer is C.

Choice	Peer answers
Severe hepatotoxicity with therapeutic doses	10%
Increased anticoagulant effects	2%
Combined central nervous system (CNS) depression decreases psychomotor performance	85%
Masked signs of delirium tremens	3%

A – Incorrect. Acetaminophen at therapeutic doses, not tricyclic antidepressants, can result in severe hepatotoxicity in chronic alcoholics.

B – Incorrect. Oral anticoagulants, not tricyclic antidepressants, can have decreased anticoagulant effects in chronic alcoholics.

C – Correct. Alcohol abuse, combined with tricyclic antidepressants such as desipramine, can result in combined CNS depression, resulting in decreased psychomotor performance, especially in the first week of treatment.

D – Incorrect. Beta-adrenergic blockers, when combined with alcohol abuse, may result in masked signs of delirium tremens.

Reference
Stahl SM, Grady MM. *Stahl's illustrated substance use and impulsive disorders.* New York, NY: Cambridge University Press; 2012. (Chapter 14)

QUESTION SEVENTEEN

A 57-year-old man presents with depression and a history of obsessive-compulsive symptoms that began in his twenties and are mostly religious in nature. He has not responded to numerous previous trials of serotonergic medications at typical depression doses. He fairly recently began cognitive behavioral therapy and has responded well to it; however, he continues to experience significant symptoms of obsessive-compulsive disorder (OCD), rating his symptoms a 7/10 in severity. His current medications include fluoxetine 80 mg/day and trazodone 50 mg/night. Which of the following is true regarding the appropriate dosing of selective serotonin reuptake inhibitors (SSRIs) in OCD?

A. Doses are typically lower than those in depression

B. Doses are typically the same as those in depression

C. Doses are typically higher than those in depression

Answer to Question Seventeen

The correct answer is C.

Choice	Peer answers
Doses are typically lower than those in depression	5%
Doses are typically the same as those in depression	3%
Doses are typically higher than those in depression	92%

A – Incorrect.

B – Incorrect.

C – Correct. Higher doses of SSRIs than those used in depression are often needed in OCD, in many cases exceeding the recommended maximum dose.

Recommended daily doses for OCD	
Citalopram	40 mg*
Clomipramine	250 mg
Escitalopram	60 mg
Fluoxetine	120 mg
Fluvoxamine	450 mg
Paroxetine	100 mg
Sertraline	400 mg

*The previous recommended daily dose for citalopram in OCD was 120 mg/day; however, the label for citalopram now includes a warning that citalopram may cause QTc prolongation at doses above 40 mg/day.

Reference

Abudy A, Juven-Wetzler A, Zohar J. Pharmacological management of treatment-resistant obsessive-compulsive disorder. *CNS Drugs* 2011;25(7):585–96.

QUESTION EIGHTEEN

Robin is a 31-year-old patient with a history of OCD being treated with cognitive behavioral therapy. She is currently 3 months pregnant, and the severity of her obsessions and compulsions has increased during her pregnancy. Which pharmacotherapy would be the preferred option for Robin?

A. Clonazepam

B. Clomipramine

C. Paroxetine

D. Fluoxetine

E. Sertraline

Answer to Question Eighteen

The correct answer is E.

Choice	Peer answers
Clonazepam	1%
Clomipramine	3%
Paroxetine	3%
Fluoxetine	16%
Sertraline	76%

The decision regarding treatment regimen for OCD in women during pregnancy is very difficult. The decision must be based on several factors, such as the risks of untreated maternal psychiatric illness and the known or unknown potential effects of psychotropic medications, benefits of pharmacological treatment, and alternative treatments to medication. Decision-making requires detailed psychiatric assessment including individual and family history of psychiatric disorders, side effects or therapeutic effects of medications, severity of disorder, and degree of impairment in occupational, family, and social areas secondary to the disorder. All steps of the treatment should be administered in agreement with the patient and her relatives. If the patient has severe depression and anxiety symptoms, a high suicide risk, considerable feeding and sleep disturbances secondary to OCD, or has mild to moderate OCD that is unresponsive to cognitive behavioral therapy, pharmacological treatment regimens may be considered.

A – Incorrect. Clonazepam is generally not effective for OCD. Additionally, exposure to any type of benzodiazepine during the first 3 months of pregnancy should be avoided.

B – Incorrect. In the general population, clomipramine is a first-line agent to treat OCD. However, several studies have suggested an approximately twofold increased risk of congenital cardiovascular defects associated with clomipramine. In addition, the risk of maternal intolerance is relatively high, and the risk for poor neonatal adaptation syndrome (PNAS) is high.

C and D – Incorrect. Paroxetine and fluoxetine are not the best first-line choice because these drugs are the most frequently associated with congenital malformations and PNAS. Data suggest that some birth defects occur 2–3.5 times more frequently among the infants of women treated with paroxetine or fluoxetine early in pregnancy.

E – Correct. An SSRI is the recommended first-line option for the treatment of OCD during pregnancy with adequate risk–benefit assessment. Sertraline is reported to be most effective in OCD but has the least number of studies focusing on the association with birth defects. The use of pharmacotherapy in moderate to severe OCD must be carefully weighed. As a general rule, the dose of any drug should be as low as possible during pregnancy.

References

Marchesi C, Ossola P, Amerio A et al. Clinical management of perinatal anxiety disorders: a systematic review. *J Affect Disord* 2016;190:543–50.

Myles N, Newall H, Ward H, Large M. Systematic meta-analysis of individual selective serotonin reuptake inhibitor medications and congenital malformations. *Aust N Z J Psychiatry* 2013;47:1002–12.

Ram D, Gandotra S. Antidepressants, anxiolytics, and hypnotics in pregnancy and lactation. *Indian J Psychiatry* 2015;57(Suppl 2):S354–71.

Reefhuis J, Devine O, Friedman JM, Louik C, Honein MA. Specific SSRIs and birth defects: Bayesian analysis to interpret new data in the context of previous reports. *BMJ* 2015;351:h3190.

QUESTION NINETEEN

A 19-year-old male in his first year of college is seeking help for possible attention deficit hyperactivity disorder (ADHD). Evaluation of the patient suggests a diagnosis of ADHD may be warranted, but there is some concern that he is drug seeking. Therefore, when selecting a treatment, his care provider takes into account the fact that self-reported "high" for stimulants correlates with:

A. Changes in extracellular dopamine

B. Changes in intracellular dopamine

C. Drug plasma levels

D. Rate of drug delivery to the brain

STAHL'S SELF-ASSESSMENT EXAMINATION IN PSYCHIATRY

Substance Use/Impulsive-Compulsive Disorders and Their Treatment

Answer to Question Nineteen

The correct answer is D.

Choice	Peer answers
Changes in extracellular dopamine	14%
Changes in intracellular dopamine	11%
Drug plasma levels	9%
Rate of drug delivery to the brain	66%

A and B – Incorrect. Acute drug use causes dopamine release in the striatum. However, the reinforcing effects of the drug are largely determined not only by the presence of dopamine, but also by the rate at which dopamine increases in the brain, which in turn is dictated by the speed at which the drug enters and leaves the brain.

C – Incorrect. Drug plasma levels in and of themselves do not determine the rate at which the drug enters the brain and causes an increase in dopamine levels.

D – Correct. Reinforcing effects of a drug are determined largely by the speed at which the drug causes an increase in dopamine in the brain. This is likely because abrupt and large increases in dopamine (such as those caused by drugs of abuse) mimic the phasic dopamine firing associated with conveying information about reward and saliency. Research shows that the self-reported high associated with intravenous (IV) cocaine use correlates with both the rate and extent of dopamine transporter (DAT) blockade. The rate of drug uptake is subject to the route of administration, with IV administration and inhalation producing the fastest drug uptake, followed by snorting. In addition, different drugs of abuse have different "reward values" (i.e., different rates at which they increase dopamine) based on their individual mechanisms of action.

References

Stahl SM. *Stahl's essential psychopharmacology*, fifth edition. New York, NY: Cambridge University Press; 2021.

Stahl SM, Grady MM. *Stahl's illustrated substance use and impulsive disorders*. New York, NY: Cambridge University Press; 2012.

CHAPTER PEER COMPARISON

For the Substance Use/Impulsive-Compulsive Disorders section, the correct answer was selected 73% of the time.

10 UNIPOLAR DEPRESSION AND ITS TREATMENT

QUESTION ONE

A 26-year-old woman began treatment for a major depressive episode 8 months ago. Two months into her treatment she began to experience noticeable symptom improvement, and for the last 5 months she has been mostly symptom free, except for persistent cognitive dysfunction. Which of the following statements regarding cognitive dysfunction in depression is most accurate?

A. Cognitive dysfunction is one of the most common residual symptoms following recovery

B. Cognitive dysfunction can be treated with serotonergic modulation of glutamate transmission

C. Both A and B

Answer to Question One

The correct answer is C.

Choice	Peer answers
Cognitive dysfunction is one of the most common residual symptoms following recovery	14%
Cognitive dysfunction can be treated with serotonergic modulation of glutamate transmission	6%
Both A and B	81%

A – Partially correct.

B – Partially correct.

C – Correct. Cognitive dysfunction is one of the most common residual symptoms of major depressive disorder and can endure longer than mood symptoms following recovery. Moreover, cognitive dysfunction is strongly correlated with physical, mental, and functional disability. Pharmacotherapies used to treat depression that have action on glutamate signaling via serotonergic modulation also show pro-cognitive effects. The prime example is vortioxetine, which has agonist action at 5HT1A, weak partial agonist action at 5HT1B/D, and antagonist action at 5HT3, 5HT1D, 5HT7, and the serotonin transporter. Antagonism of 5HT3 disinhibits glutamate release, while antagonism of 5HT7 enhances release of glutamate release in the prefrontal cortex. In addition, agonism of 5HT1A (full) and 5HT1B (partial) may enhance or suppress glutamate transmission based on neuronal localization.

References

Pehrson AL, Sanchez C. Serotonergic modulation of glutamate neurotransmission as a strategy for treating depression and cognitive dysfunction. *CNS Spectr* 2014;19(2):121–33.

Rock PL, Roiser JP, Riedel WJ, Blackwell AD. Cognitive impairment in depression: a systematic review and meta-analysis. *Psychol Med* 2014;44(10):2029–40.

Zajecka JM. Residual symptoms and relapse: mood, cognitive symptoms, and sleep disturbances. *J Clin Psychiatry* 2013;74(Suppl 2):9–13.

Zuckerman H, Pan Z, Park C et al. Recognition and treatment of cognitive dysfunction in major depressive disorder. *Front Psychiatry* 2018;9:655.

QUESTION TWO

Amir is a 19-year-old patient with depression. He requests treatment with a serotonin norepinephrine reuptake inhibitor (SNRI) because he heard they are more effective than selective serotonin reuptake inhibitors (SSRIs). Theoretically, what is the therapeutic advantage of an SNRI over an SSRI?

A. Increased norepinephrine via norepinephrine transporter inhibition

B. Increased dopamine via norepinephrine transporter inhibition

C. Increased norepinephrine and dopamine via norepinephrine transporter inhibition

Answer to Question Two

The correct answer is C.

Choice	Peer answers
Increased norepinephrine via norepinephrine transporter inhibition	31%
Increased dopamine via norepinephrine transporter inhibition	3%
Increased norepinephrine and dopamine via norepinephrine transporter inhibition	66%

A – Partially correct.

B – Partially correct.

C – Correct. In addition to boosting serotonin like SSRIs (via inhibition of serotonin reuptake by the serotonin transporter [SERT]), SNRIs can boost norepinephrine by inhibiting reuptake by the norepinephrine transporter (NET). Additionally, in the prefrontal cortex, SNRIs can boost dopamine levels. In the prefrontal cortex, SERTs and NETs are present in abundance on serotonin and norepinephrine nerve terminals, respectively, but there are very few dopamine transporters (DATs) on dopamine nerve terminals. Therefore, dopamine action is terminated by either enzymatic degradation or NET. If NET is inhibited by an SNRI then it cannot terminate the action of dopamine and dopamine levels increase in this brain region.

References

Ranjbar-Slamloo Y, **Fazlali Z**. Dopamine and noradrenaline in the brain; overlapping or dissociate functions? *Front Mol Neurosci* 2020;12:334.

Stahl SM. *Stahl's essential psychopharmacology*, fifth edition. New York, NY: Cambridge University Press; 2021. (Chapter 7)

QUESTION THREE

A 36-year-old man with major depressive disorder is having lab work done to assess his levels of inflammatory markers. Based on the current evidence regarding inflammation in depression, which of the following results would you most likely suspect for this patient?

A. Elevated levels of tumor necrosis factor-alpha (TNF-α)

B. Reduced levels of interleukin 6 (IL-6)

C. Reduced C-reactive protein (CRP)

D. Elevated interferon gamma (IFNγ)

Unipolar Depression and Its Treatment

Answer to Question Three

The correct answer is A.

Choice	Peer answers
Elevated levels of tumor necrosis factor-alpha (TNF-α)	65%
Reduced levels of interleukin 6 (IL-6)	10%
Reduced C-reactive protein (CRP)	12%
Elevated interferon gamma (IFNγ)	13%

A – Correct. There is growing evidence that inflammation may play an important role in the pathophysiology of major depression. Clinical studies have shown that depressed patients have significantly higher concentrations of several inflammatory central and peripheral markers, including the pro-inflammatory cytokines TNF-α and IL-6. Patients with depression also have higher concentrations of CRP, which is synthesized by the liver in response to pro-inflammatory cytokines, and reduced IFNγ, which is a pro-inflammatory cytokine. Furthermore, both cytokines and cytokine inducers can cause symptoms of depression. For example, as many as 50% of patients receiving chronic therapy with the cytokine interferon develop symptoms consistent with idiopathic depression.

B, C, and D – Incorrect.

References

Enache D, Pariante CM, Mondelli V. Markers of central inflammation in major depressive disorder: a systematic review and meta-analysis of studies examining cerebrospinal fluid, positron emission tomography and post-mortem brain tissue. *Brain Behav Immun* 2019;81:24–40.

Haapakoski R, Mathieu J, Ebmeier KP, Alenius H, Kivimäki M. Cumulative meta-analysis of interleukins 6 and 1β, tumour necrosis factor α and C-reactive protein in patients with major depressive disorder. *Brain Behav Immun* 2015;49:206–15.

Köhler CA, Freitas TH, Maes M et al. Peripheral cytokine and chemokine alterations in depression: a meta-analysis of 82 studies. *Acta Psychiatr Scand* 2017;135(5):373–87.

Raison CL, Miller AH. Is depression an inflammatory disorder? *Curr Psychiatry Rep* 2011;13:467–75.

QUESTION FOUR

A 28-year-old man with moderate depression achieves remission after 16 weeks on a therapeutic dose of an antidepressant. According to the neurotrophic hypothesis of depression, which of the following is most likely true of his brain-derived neurotrophic factor (BDNF) expression before and after his successful treatment?

A. BDNF expression was abnormally low while he was depressed, and increased during antidepressant treatment

B. BDNF expression was abnormally high while he was depressed, and decreased during antidepressant treatment

C. BDNF expression was normal while he was depressed, and was unaffected during antidepressant treatment

Unipolar Depression and Its Treatment

Answer to Question Four

The correct answer is A.

Choice	Peer answers
BDNF expression was abnormally low while he was depressed, and increased during antidepressant treatment	89%
BDNF expression was abnormally high while he was depressed, and decreased during antidepressant treatment	10%
BDNF expression was normal while he was depressed, and was unaffected during antidepressant treatment	1%

A – Correct. The neurotrophic hypothesis of depression posits that depression results from decreased neurotrophic support, leading to neuronal atrophy, decreased hippocampal neurogenesis, and that antidepressant treatment blocks or reverses this deficit, thereby reversing atrophy and cell loss. Several meta-analyses have reported deficient BDNF levels in patients with major depressive disorder and an elevation in BDNF following antidepressant treatment.

B – Incorrect.

C – Incorrect.

References
Polyakova M, Stuke K, Schuemberg K et al. BDNF as a biomarker for successful treatment of mood disorders: a systematic & quantitative meta-analysis. *J Affect Disord* 2015;174:432–40.

Sen S, Duman R, Sanacora G. Serum brain-derived neurotrophic factor, depression, and antidepressant medications: meta-analyses and implications. *Biol Psychiatry* 2008;64(6):527–32.

Zhou C, Zhong J, Zou B et al. Meta-analyses of comparative efficacy of antidepressant medications on peripheral BDNF concentration in patients with depression. *PLoS One* 2017;12(2):e0172270.

QUESTION FIVE

Margaret is a 42-year-old patient with untreated depression. She is reluctant to begin antidepressant treatment due to concerns about treatment-induced weight gain. Which of the following antidepressant treatments is associated with the greatest risk of weight gain?

A. Escitalopram

B. Fluoxetine

C. Mirtazapine

D. Vilazodone

Answer to Question Five

The correct answer is C.

Choice	Peer answers
Escitalopram	2%
Fluoxetine	4%
Mirtazapine	93%
Vilazodone	1%

A – Incorrect. Although weight gain may occur, it is not commonly reported with escitalopram, and a meta-analysis suggests that the risk of both short- and long-term weight gain with escitalopram is low.

B – Incorrect. Although weight gain may occur, it is not commonly reported with fluoxetine and a meta-analysis did not find significant increase in weight over the short or long term. Some patients actually experience short-term weight loss with fluoxetine.

C – Correct. Meta-analysis has shown that mirtazapine, an alpha 2 antagonist, may cause both short- and long-term weight gain. This is consistent with its secondary pharmacological properties: mirtazapine is an antagonist at both serotonin 2C and histamine 1 receptors, the combination of which has been proposed to cause weight gain. However, it should be noted that average weight gain with any antidepressant is small, and rather than a widespread effect it may instead be that a small number of individuals experience significant weight gain due to their genetic predispositions and other factors.

D – Incorrect. Although weight gain may occur, studies with vilazodone have suggested a lower risk for weight gain compared to many other antidepressants that block serotonin reuptake; however, head-to-head studies have not been conducted.

References

Serretti A, Mandelli L. Antidepressants and body weight: a comprehensive review and meta-analysis. *J Clin Psychiatry* 2010;71(10):1259–72.

Stahl SM. *Stahl's essential psychopharmacology, the prescriber's guide*, seventh edition. New York, NY: Cambridge University Press; 2020.

QUESTION SIX

A 52-year-old man presents to the emergency room with symptoms of hypertensive crisis after an evening dining out with friends. He is currently taking a monoamine oxidase inhibitor (MAOI). Which of the following foods must be avoided by patients taking MAOIs?

A. Fresh fish

B. Aged cheese

C. Bananas

D. Bottled beer

Answer to Question Six

The correct answer is B.

Choice	Peer answers
Fresh fish	0%
Aged cheese	98%
Bananas	0%
Bottled beer	2%

Tyramine content in food can instigate a hypertensive crisis in patients taking MAOIs. Meals considered to contain a high level of tyramine content generally include 40 mg of tyramine.

Foods to AVOID*	Foods ALLOWED
Dried, aged, smoked, fermented, spoiled, or improperly stored meat, poultry, and fish	Fresh or processed meat, poultry, and fish
Broad bean pods	All other vegetables
Aged cheeses	Processed cheese slices, cottage cheese, ricotta cheese, cream cheese, yogurt
Tap and unpasteurized beer	Bottled or canned beer and alcohol
Marmite	Brewer's and baker's yeast
Soy products/tofu	Peanuts
Banana peel	Bananas, avocados, raspberries
Sauerkraut, kimchee	
Tyramine-containing nutritional supplements	

*Not necessary for 6-mg transdermal or low-dose oral selegiline.

A – Incorrect. Fresh fish does not have a high tyramine content and can therefore be safely consumed when one is taking an MAOI.

B – Correct. Aged cheeses in general have high tyramine content and must be avoided when a patient is taking an MAOI.

C – Incorrect. Bananas that are not overripe do not have a high tyramine content and can therefore be safely consumed when one is taking an MAOI. However, banana peels and bananas that are overripe should be avoided.

D – Incorrect. Bottled beer does not have a high tyramine content and can therefore be safely consumed when one is taking an MAOI.

Reference

Gillman PK. A reassessment of the safety profile of monoamine oxidase inhibitors: elucidating tired old tyramine myths. *J Neural Transm (Vienna)* 2018;125(11):1707–17.

Unipolar Depression and Its Treatment

QUESTION SEVEN

A 48-year-old woman with a history of treatment-resistant depression is currently taking duloxetine 60 mg/day with partial response as well as trazodone 50 mg/day for insomnia. Despite reporting strict adherence to her medication dosages, she states that she feels empty and useless, and she admits to having thoughts of death. She states that she does not have plans to kill herself because it would harm her family and pets. Her clinician decides to try tranylcypromine, a monoamine oxidase inhibitor (MAOI) and one of the few agents that she has not yet tried. Which of the patient's current medications MUST you discontinue BEFORE initiating tranylcypromine?

A. Duloxetine

B. Trazodone

C. Both duloxetine and trazodone

D. Neither duloxetine nor trazodone

Answer to Question Seven

The correct answer is A.

Choice	Peer answers
Duloxetine	51%
Trazodone	4%
Both duloxetine and trazodone	43%
Neither duloxetine nor trazodone	2%

A – Correct. Duloxetine is a serotonin norepinephrine reuptake inhibitor. Inhibition of the serotonin transporter leads to increased synaptic availability of serotonin. Similarly, inhibition of MAO leads to increased serotonin levels. In combination, these two mechanisms can cause excessive stimulation of postsynaptic serotonin receptors, which has the potential to cause a fatal "serotonin syndrome" or "serotonin toxicity." Because of the risk of serotonin toxicity, complete washout of duloxetine is necessary before starting an MAOI. Duloxetine must be down-titrated as tolerated, after which one must wait five half-lives of duloxetine (at least 3–4 days) before initiating the MAOI.

B – Incorrect. Although trazodone does have serotonin reuptake inhibition at antidepressant doses (150 mg or higher), this property is not clinically relevant at the low doses used for insomnia. In fact, because there is a required gap in antidepressant treatment when switching to or from an MAOI, low-dose trazodone can be useful as a bridging agent when switching.

C and D – Incorrect.

References

Dvir Y, Smallwood P. Serotonin syndrome: a complex but easily avoidable condition. *Gen Hosp Psychiatry* 2008;30(3):284–7.

Stahl SM. *Stahl's essential psychopharmacology, the prescriber's guide*, seventh edition. New York, NY: Cambridge University Press; 2020.

Wimbiscus M, Kostenkjo O, Malone D. MAO inhibitors: risks, benefits, and lore. *Cleve Clin J Med* 2010;77(12):859–82.

Unipolar Depression and Its Treatment

QUESTION EIGHT

A 56-year-old male patient with major depression is brought to the emergency room with cardiac arrhythmia and possible cardiac arrest. While at the hospital, he suffers a seizure. His wife states that he may have ingested an increased dose of his medication. Which of the following is most likely responsible for this apparent overdose reaction?

A. Atomoxetine

B. Clomipramine

C. Fluvoxamine

D. Venlafaxine

Answer to Question Eight

The correct answer is B.

Choice	Peer answers
Atomoxetine	7%
Clomipramine	77%
Fluvoxamine	3%
Venlafaxine	12%

A – Incorrect. Atomoxetine, a norepinephrine reuptake inhibitor, does not block voltage-sensitive sodium channels (VSSCs) and is not noted to have severe cardiac impairments upon overdose; rather sedation, agitation, hyperactivity, abnormal behavior, and gastrointestinal symptoms are most commonly reported.

B – Correct. Clomipramine, a tricyclic antidepressant (TCA), may be most likely to cause these effects in overdose. TCAs block VSSCs in both the brain and the heart. This action is weak at therapeutic doses, but in overdose may lead to coma, seizures, and cardiac arrhythmia, and may even prove fatal.

C – Incorrect. Fluvoxamine, a selective serotonin reuptake inhibitor (SSRI), also does not block VSSCs and does not generally cause severe cardiac impairment in overdose.

D – Incorrect. Venlafaxine is a serotonin norepinephrine reuptake inhibitor (SNRI). Although some data have suggested that SNRIs can affect heart function in overdose and also may carry increased risk of death in overdose compared to SSRIs, their toxicity in overdose is less than that for TCAs.

References

Stahl SM. *Stahl's essential psychopharmacology*, fifth edition. New York, NY: Cambridge University Press; 2021. (Chapter 7)

Thanacoody HK, Thomas SH. Tricyclic antidepressant poisoning: cardiovascular toxicity. *Toxicol Rev* 2005;24(3):205–14.

QUESTION NINE

A 65-year-old patient on theophylline for chronic obstructive pulmonary disease (COPD) and fluvoxamine for recurring depressive episodes required a decreased dose of theophylline due to increased blood levels of the drug. Which of the following pharmacokinetic properties may be responsible for this?

A. Inhibition of CYP450 1A2 by fluvoxamine

B. Inhibition of CYP450 2D6 by fluvoxamine

C. Inhibition of CYP450 3A4 by fluvoxamine

Answer to Question Nine

The correct answer is A.

Choice	Peer answers
Inhibition of CYP450 1A2 by fluvoxamine	48%
Inhibition of CYP450 2D6 by fluvoxamine	37%
Inhibition of CYP450 3A4 by fluvoxamine	16%

A – Correct. Fluvoxamine is a strong inhibitor of CYP450 1A2. The-ophylline is metabolized in part by CYP450 1A2, and thus strong inhibition of this enzyme by fluvoxamine may require a dose reduction of theophylline if the two are given concomitantly, so as to avoid increased blood levels of the drug.

B – Incorrect. Of all selective serotonin reuptake inhibitors (SSRIs), fluvoxamine shows the least interaction with CYP450 2D6.

C – Incorrect. Fluvoxamine is also a moderate inhibitor of CYP450 3A4, but since theophylline is neither a substrate nor an inhibitor of 3A4, this should not affect theophylline blood levels.

References

Stahl SM. *Stahl's essential psychopharmacology, the prescriber's guide*, seventh edition. New York, NY: Cambridge University Press; 2020.

Stahl SM. *Stahl's essential psychopharmacology*, fifth edition. New York, NY: Cambridge University Press; 2021. (Chapter 7)

QUESTION TEN

Mike, a 31-year-old patient with major depressive disorder (MDD), has experienced some response with the serotonin norepinephrine reuptake inhibitor (SNRI) venlafaxine XR (150 mg/day). However, the patient acknowledges that he and his wife have been having relationship problems because of his poor libido. The patient experienced this problem prior to being diagnosed and treated for MDD, but he has found that the venlafaxine has worsened this troubling symptom despite the fact that his mood has improved. He asks if there is a way to both prevent worsening of his mood and avoid this side effect. Which of the following treatment strategies would you recommend for this patient?

A. Decrease venlafaxine dose

B. Switch to a norepinephrine and dopamine reuptake inhibitor (NDRI)

C. Switch to a selective serotonin reuptake inhibitor (SSRI)

D. Augment current venlafaxine dose with a phosphodiesterase-5 inhibitor (e.g., sildenafil)

Answer to Question Ten

The correct answer is B.

Choice	Peer answers
Decrease venlafaxine dose	5%
Switch to a norepinephrine and dopamine reuptake inhibitor (NDRI)	64%
Switch to a selective serotonin reuptake inhibitor (SSRI)	2%
Augment current venlafaxine dose with a phosphodiesterase-5 inhibitor (e.g., sildenafil)	29%

The prevalence of sexual dysfunction, including diminished libido, impaired arousal, and lack of orgasm, is high among patients with MDD, and sexual dysfunction may worsen with antidepressant treatment (particularly treatment with a serotonin reuptake inhibitor). Serotonin plays an inhibitory role in the human sexual response, both for desire and for orgasm. Exacerbation of sexual dysfunction by antidepressant treatment is one of the most common factors reported to cause treatment nonadherence or discontinuation.

A – Incorrect. With regards to the diagnostic criteria for depression, this patient has experienced some improvement with his current dose of venlafaxine. Although lowering the dose of venlafaxine may improve this patient's sexual function, a dose reduction may also increase his depressive symptoms.

B – Correct. Pharmacological agents that increase dopaminergic neurotransmission and/or decrease serotonergic neurotransmission (e.g., serotonin 1A agonists or serotonin 2 antagonists) are often effective in ameliorating sexual dysfunction. Switching to an NDRI such as bupropion would be expected to increase dopaminergic neurotransmission and improve sexual function. Given that the patient experienced libido problems prior to treatment with the SNRI, and that the problem has worsened on treatment with the SNRI, it makes sense to switch to bupropion. *Augmentation* with bupropion to address sexual dysfunction, although commonly done in clinical practice, is not actually supported by randomized controlled studies.

C – Incorrect. Of the available antidepressant treatments, SSRIs are associated with the greatest risk of worsening sexual function, so switching from venlafaxine to an SSRI would not be expected to improve sexual functioning.

D – Incorrect. Although it is usually best to try another antidepressant monotherapy before resorting to augmentation strategies for the treatment of side effects, for a patient such as this who is otherwise responding well it might be reasonable to augment. However, phosphodiesterase-5 inhibitors do not increase desire and thus would not be a good option to treat this patient's specific problems with sexual function.

References

Kennedy SH, Rizvi S. Sexual dysfunction, depression, and the impact of antidepressants. *J Clin Psychopharmacol* 2009;29(2):157–64.

Serretti A, Chiesa A. Sexual side effects of pharmacological treatment of psychiatric diseases. *Clin Pharmacol Ther* 2011;89(1):142–7.

Unipolar Depression and Its Treatment

QUESTION ELEVEN

In addition to treating depressed mood, preclinical data indicate that serotonin 5HT3 receptor antagonists may have clinical utility as adjunct treatment for which symptoms?

A. Cognitive symptoms

B. Irritability

C. Psychomotor retardation

D. Sleep problems

Answer to Question Eleven

The correct answer is A.

Choice	Peer answers
Cognitive symptoms	74%
Irritability	5%
Psychomotor retardation	5%
Sleep problems	15%

A – Correct. Serotonergic neurons synapse with noradrenergic neurons, cholinergic neurons, and GABAergic interneurons, all of which contain serotonin 5HT3 receptors. When serotonin is released, it binds to 5HT3 receptors on GABAergic neurons, which release gamma-aminobutyric acid (GABA) onto noradrenergic, glutamatergic, and cholinergic neurons, thus reducing release of norepinephrine, glutamate, and acetylcholine, respectively. In addition, serotonin may bind to 5HT3 receptors on noradrenergic and cholinergic neurons, further reducing release of those neurotransmitters. This may theoretically contribute to symptoms of depressed mood and impaired cognition. Therefore, treatment with 5HT3 receptor antagonists improves depressed mood and cognitive problems.

B, C, and D – Incorrect. Irritability, psychomotor retardation, and sleep problems are not associated with antagonism at 5HT3 receptors.

References

Artigas F. Serotonin receptors involved in antidepressant effects. *Pharmacol Ther* 2013;137:119–31.

Carr GV, Lucki I. The role of serotonin receptor subtypes in treating depression: a review of animal studies. *Psychopharmacology* 2011;213:265–8.

Ciranna L. Serotonin as a modulator of glutamate- and GABA-mediated neurotransmission: implications in physiological functions and in pathology. *Curr Neuropharmacol* 2006;4(2):101–14.

Pehrson AL, Sanchez C. Serotonergic modulation of glutamate neurotransmission as a strategy for treating depression and cognitive dysfunction. *CNS Spectr* 2014;19(2):121–33.

Unipolar Depression and Its Treatment

QUESTION TWELVE

A 36-year-old patient has only partially responded to his second monotherapy with a first-line antidepressant. Which of the following has the best evidence of efficacy for augmenting antidepressants in patients with inadequate response?

A. Adding an atypical antipsychotic

B. Adding buspirone

C. Adding a stimulant

Answer to Question Twelve

The correct answer is A.

Choice	Peer answers
Adding an atypical antipsychotic	86%
Adding buspirone	12%
Adding a stimulant	1%

A – Correct. Atypical antipsychotics have been studied as adjuncts to selective serotonin reuptake inhibitors (SSRIs) and serotonin norepinephrine reuptake inhibitors (SNRIs), with approvals for aripiprazole, brexpiprazole, quetiapine XR, and olanzapine (in combination with fluoxetine). Overall, most studies of atypical antipsychotics show a benefit of combination treatment over monotherapy, although effect sizes have been modest. Although atypical antipsychotics have the best evidence of efficacy for augmenting antidepressants in patients with inadequate response, their adverse event profiles may still put them later in the treatment algorithm.

B – Incorrect. Although adding buspirone, a serotonin 1A partial agonist, to a first-line antidepressant makes sense mechanistically, the limited data that exist are mixed/weak.

C – Incorrect. The limited controlled data for stimulant augmentation in depression show a trend of benefit; however, this strategy is not as well documented as is augmentation with atypical antipsychotics.

References

Bech P, Fava M, Trivedi MH, Wisniewski SR, Rush AJ. Outcomes on the pharmacopsychometric triangle in bupropion-SR vs. buspirone augmentation of citalopram in the STAR*D trial. *Acta Psychiatr Scand* 2012;125(4):342–8.

Citrome L. Adjunctive aripiprazole, olanzapine, or quetiapine for major depressive disorder: an analysis of number needed to treat, number needed to harm, and likelihood to be helped or harmed. *Postgrad Med* 2010;122(4):39–48.

Trivedi MH, Cutler AJ, Richards C et al. A randomized controlled trial of the efficacy and safety of lisdexamfetamine dimesylate as augmentation therapy in adults with residual symptoms of major depressive disorder after treatment with escitalopram. *J Clin Psychiatry* 2013;74(8):802–9.

Zhou X, Ravindran AV, Qin B, et al. Comparative efficacy, acceptability, and tolerability of augmentation agents in treatment-resistant depression: systematic review and network meta-analysis. *J Clin Psychiatry* 2015;76(4):e487–98.

Unipolar Depression and Its Treatment

QUESTION THIRTEEN

Miryam is a 24-year-old woman with a major depressive episode that is only partially responding to treatment with a selective serotonin reuptake inhibitor. In particular, she continues to display reduced positive affect. She is prescribed adjunctive bupropion to manage this symptom. Through which mechanism(s) does bupropion theoretically ameliorate reduced positive affect?

A. Inhibition of the serotonin transporter

B. Inhibition of the dopamine transporter

C. Inhibition of the norepinephrine transporter

D. A and B

E. A and C

F. B and C

Answer to Question Thirteen

The correct answer is F.

Choice	Peer answers
Inhibition of the serotonin transporter	2%
Inhibition of the dopamine transporter	6%
Inhibition of the norepinephrine transporter	4%
A and B	4%
A and C	4%
B and C	80%

A – Incorrect. Bupropion does not appear to have pharmacological action on the serotonin transporter.

B, C, D, and E – Partially correct.

F – Correct. Bupropion has weak reuptake blocking properties for dopamine (dopamine transporter [DAT] inhibition), and for norepinephrine (norepinephrine transporter [NET] inhibition). Human positron emission tomography scans suggest that as little as 10–15% and perhaps no more than 20–30% of striatal DATs may be occupied at therapeutic doses of bupropion. NET occupancy would be expected to be in this same range.

References

Nutt D, Demyttenaere K, Janka Z et al. The other face of depression, reduced positive affect: the role of catecholamines in causation and cure. *J Psychopharmacol* 2007;21(5):461–71.

Stahl SM. *Stahl's essential psychopharmacology*, fifth edition. New York, NY: Cambridge University Press; 2021. (Chapter 7)

Tomarken AJ, Dichter GS, Freid C, Addington S, Shelton RC. Assessing the effects of bupropion SR on mood dimensions of depression. *J Affect Disord* 2004;78(3):235–41.

QUESTION FOURTEEN

Wei is a 33-year-old patient with major depressive disorder beginning at age 17; his current depressive episode has persisted for 10 months. His treatment history includes fluoxetine, nefazodone, venlafaxine, mirtazapine, agomelatine, lithium augmentation, and electroconvulsive therapy. Each of these treatments produced moderate but transient response; therefore, he will begin ketamine infusions to treat his treatment-resistant depression. Which of the following statements about ketamine treatment is true?

A. The strongest evidence for the efficacy of ketamine is in bipolar depression

B. Repeated dosing extends the duration of ketamine effects

C. High-frequency ketamine administration is recommended

D. A history of antidepressant treatment is not necessary to start ketamine treatment

Answer to Question Fourteen

The correct answer is B.

Choice	Peer answers
The strongest evidence for the efficacy of ketamine is in bipolar depression	8%
Repeated dosing extends the duration of ketamine effects	74%
High-frequency ketamine administration is recommended	12%
A history of antidepressant treatment is not necessary to start ketamine treatment	7%

A – Incorrect. To date, the strongest evidence for ketamine's clinical benefit in psychiatric disorders is in the treatment of major depressive episodes without psychotic features associated with major depressive disorder.

B – Correct. Studies suggest that repeated dosing may extend the duration of ketamine effects. Ketamine administration of 2–3 times per week over 2–3 weeks, followed by a taper period and/or continued treatments may be most effective.

C – Incorrect. High-frequency ketamine administration is not recommended. Chronic high-frequency use of ketamine is associated with cognitive impairment and cystitis.

D – Incorrect. A thorough history of antidepressant treatment should be collected and documented to confirm previous adequate trials of antidepressant treatments and confirm treatment resistance.

Reference

Sanacora G, Frye MA, McDonald W et al. A consensus statement on the use of ketamine in the treatment of mood disorders. *JAMA Psychiatry* 2017;74(4):399–405.

Unipolar Depression and Its Treatment

QUESTION FIFTEEN

A patient with depression is prescribed mirtazapine as adjunctive treatment to venlafaxine, a serotonin norepinephrine reuptake inhibitor. Mirtazapine acts on alpha 2 receptors to produce what effect?

A. Disinhibition of norepinephrine and serotonin release via alpha 2 agonism

B. Disinhibition of norepinephrine and dopamine release via alpha 2 agonism

C. Disinhibition of norepinephrine and serotonin release via alpha 2 antagonism

D. Disinhibition of norepinephrine and dopamine release via alpha 2 antagonism

Answer to Question Fifteen

The correct answer is C.

Choice	Peer answers
Disinhibition of norepinephrine and serotonin release via alpha 2 agonism	13%
Disinhibition of norepinephrine and dopamine release via alpha 2 agonism	11%
Disinhibition of norepinephrine and serotonin release via alpha 2 antagonism	63%
Disinhibition of norepinephrine and dopamine release via alpha 2 antagonism	13%

A – Incorrect.

B – Incorrect.

C – Correct. Norepinephrine turns off its own release via alpha 2 pre-synaptic receptors; therefore, alpha 2 antagonism with mirtazapine facilitates disinhibition of norepinephrine. Furthermore, norepinephrine migrating from a norepinephrine terminal can also turn off serotonin release via alpha 2 presynaptic heteroreceptors on serotonin neurons. Therefore, alpha 2 antagonists like mirtazapine can have a dual effect on facilitating the release of both norepinephrine and serotonin.

D – Incorrect.

References

Anttila SA, Leinonen EV. A review of the pharmacological and clinical profile of mirtazapine. *CNS Drug Rev* 2001;7(3):249–64.

Stahl SM. *Stahl's essential psychopharmacology*, fifth edition. New York, NY: Cambridge University Press; 2021. (Chapters 6, 7)

Unipolar Depression and Its Treatment

QUESTION SIXTEEN

A 34-year-old man with depression characterized by depressed mood, sleep difficulties, and concentration problems has not responded well to a selective serotonin reuptake inhibitor (SSRI) or a serotonin norepinephrine reuptake inhibitor (SNRI). His clinician elects to switch him to vortioxetine, which has prominent serotonin 5HT7 receptor antagonism. What may be a primary function of these receptors?

A. Regulation of serotonin–acetylcholine interactions

B. Regulation of serotonin–dopamine interactions

C. Regulation of serotonin–glutamate interactions

D. Regulation of serotonin–norepinephrine interactions

Answer to Question Sixteen

The correct answer is C.

Choice	Peer answers
Regulation of serotonin–acetylcholine interactions	11%
Regulation of serotonin–dopamine interactions	13%
Regulation of serotonin–glutamate interactions	69%
Regulation of serotonin–norepinephrine interactions	8%

A – Incorrect.

B – Incorrect.

C – Correct. Serotonin 5HT7 receptors are postsynaptic G-protein-linked receptors. They are localized in the cortex, hippocampus, hypothalamus, thalamus, and brainstem raphe nuclei, where they regulate mood, circadian rhythms, sleep, learning, and memory. A major function of these receptors may be to regulate serotonin–glutamate interactions.

Serotonin can both activate and inhibit glutamate release from cortical pyramidal neurons. Serotonin released from neurons in the raphe nucleus can bind to 5HT2A receptors on pyramidal glutamate neurons in the prefrontal cortex, activating glutamate release. However, serotonin also binds to 5HT1A receptors on pyramidal glutamate neurons, an action that inhibits glutamate release. Additionally, serotonin binds to 5HT7 receptors on GABA interneurons in the prefrontal cortex. This stimulates GABA release, which in turn inhibits glutamate release.

Serotonin binding at 5HT7 receptors can also inhibit its own release. That is, when serotonergic neurons in the raphe nucleus are stimulated, they release serotonin throughout the brain, including not only in the prefrontal cortex but also in the raphe itself. Serotonin can then bind to 5HT7 receptors on GABA interneurons in the raphe nucleus. This stimulates GABA release, which then turns off serotonin release.

Serotonin binding at 5HT7 receptors in the raphe inhibits serotonin release; therefore, an antagonist at this receptor would be expected to enhance serotonin release. Specifically, by blocking serotonin from binding to the 5HT7 receptor on GABA interneurons, a 5HT7 antagonist would prevent the release of GABA onto serotonin neurons, thus allowing the continued release of serotonin in the prefrontal cortex.

D – Incorrect.

References
Sarkisyan G, Roberts AJ, Hedlund PB. The 5-HT$_7$ receptor as a mediator and modulator of antidepressant-like behavior. *Behav Brain Res* 2010;209(1):99–108.

Stahl SM. The serotonin-7 receptor as a novel therapeutic target. *J Clin Psychiatry* 2010;71(11):1414–15.

Unipolar Depression and Its Treatment

QUESTION SEVENTEEN

A 32-year-old woman with major depressive disorder has been taking a selective serotonin reuptake inhibitor (SSRI) with good response for months. She presents now with complaints that she feels numb, and that even when she's sad she can't cry. Her clinician is considering reducing the dose of her SSRI in an effort to alleviate this problem. Is this a reasonable option?

A. Yes, data suggest that SSRI-induced indifference is dose-dependent and can be alleviated by reducing the dose

B. No, although data suggest that SSRI-induced indifference is dose-dependent, patients who develop this side effect generally require switch to a different medication

C. No, SSRI-induced indifference is not dose-dependent and thus cannot be alleviated by reducing the dose

Unipolar Depression and Its Treatment

Answer to Question Seventeen

The correct answer is A.

Choice	Peer answers
Yes, data suggest that SSRI-induced indifference is dose-dependent and can be alleviated by reducing the dose	71%
No, although data suggest that SSRI-induced indifference is dose-dependent, patients who develop this side effect generally require switch to a different medication	22%
No, SSRI-induced indifference is not dose-dependent and thus cannot be alleviated by reducing the dose	7%

A – Correct. Apathy and emotional blunting can be symptoms of depression, but they are also side effects associated with SSRIs. These symptoms – termed "SSRI-induced indifference" – are under-recognized but can be very distressing for patients. They are theoretically due to an increase in serotonin levels and a consequent reduction of dopamine release. The first recommended strategy for addressing SSRI-induced indifference is to lower the SSRI dose, if feasible. Additional options include adding an augmenting agent or switching to an antidepressant in another class.

B and C – Incorrect.

References
Sansone RA, Sansone LA. SSRI-induced indifference. *Psychiatry (Edgemont)* 2010;7(1):14–18.

Stahl SM. *Case studies: Stahl's essential psychopharmacology*. New York, NY: Cambridge University Press; 2011.

Stahl SM. *Stahl's essential psychopharmacology, the prescriber's guide*, seventh edition. New York, NY: Cambridge University Press; 2017.

Stahl SM. *Stahl's essential psychopharmacology*, fifth edition. New York, NY: Cambridge University Press; 2021. (Chapter 7)

QUESTION EIGHTEEN

A 31-year-old woman is diagnosed with severe postpartum depression 3 weeks after giving birth. Treatment with brexanolone, a positive allosteric modulator of GABA at the GABA-A receptor, ameliorated her symptoms. GABA has more recently been implicated in the neurobiology of depression. Theoretically, individuals with depression may display a lack of normal GABAergic tonic inhibition via:

A. Postsynaptic benzodiazepine-sensitive GABA-A receptors

B. Extrasynaptic benzodiazepine-insensitive GABA-A receptor

C. Both A and B

Answer to Question Eighteen

The correct answer is B.

Choice	Peer answers
Postsynaptic benzodiazepine-sensitive GABA-A receptors	23%
Extrasynaptic benzodiazepine-insensitive GABA-A receptor	32%
Both A and B	45%

A – Incorrect. Postsynaptic benzodiazepine-sensitive GABA-A receptors are thought to mediate phasic inhibition.

B – Correct. Extrasynaptic benzodiazepine-insensitive GABA-A receptor subtypes are thought to mediate tonic inhibition. Tonic inhibition may be regulated by the ambient levels of extracellular GABA molecules that have escaped presynaptic reuptake and enzymatic destruction and persist between neurotransmissions and is boosted by allosteric modulation at these sites. Thus, tonic inhibition is thought to set the overall tone and excitability of the postsynaptic neuron, and to be important for certain regulatory events such as the frequency of neuronal discharge in response to excitatory inputs. Since neuroactive steroids have antidepressant properties, this has led to the proposal that some depressed patients may have a lack of normal tonic inhibition, and thus too much excitability in some brain circuits.

Indeed, in the case of postpartum depression, it may be potentially explainable on the basis that pregnant women have high circulating and presumably brain levels of neuroactive steroids. When they deliver, there is a precipitous decline in circulating neuroactive steroid levels, hypothetically triggering the sudden onset of a major depressive episode when tonic inhibition is lost. Restoring neuroactive steroid levels – and tonic inhibition – via brexanolone may be enough for the patient to respond by reversing their depression and then having some additional time to accommodate to the lower levels of neuroactive steroids postpartum.

C – Incorrect.

References

Maguire J. Neuroactive steroids and GABAergic involvement in the neuroendocrine dysfunction associated with major depressive disorder and postpartum depression. *Front Cell Neurosci* 2019;13:83.

Meltzer-Brody S, Kanes SJ. Allopregnanolone in postpartum depression: role in pathophysiology and treatment. *Neurobiol Stress* 2020;12:100212.

Pytka K, Dziubina A, Młyniec K et al. The role of glutamatergic, GABA-ergic, and cholinergic receptors in depression and antidepressant-like effect. *Pharmacol Rep* 2016;68(2):443–50.

Unipolar Depression and Its Treatment

QUESTION NINETEEN

A 27-year-old patient who has been taking a selective serotonin reuptake inhibitor (SSRI) for depression for the last 2 years has just found out that she is 12 weeks pregnant. Cumulative data for SSRI use in pregnancy have established a small but clinically significant increase in absolute risk of:

A. Cardiovascular malformations

B. Persistent pulmonary hypertension

C. Autism spectrum disorder

D. All of the above

E. None of the above

Unipolar Depression and Its Treatment

Answer to Question Nineteen

The correct answer is E.

Choice	Peer answers
Cardiovascular malformations	17%
Persistent pulmonary hypertension	16%
Autism spectrum disorder	16%
All of the above	12%
None of the above	39%

A – Incorrect. The evidence for increased risk of first trimester major malformations with antidepressants has been limited and inconsistent. A recent large, population-based, case-control study did not identify a substantial increase in risk of cardiac malformations with SSRI use in early pregnancy after adjusting for maternal underlying condition. Furthermore, a recent review of 22 meta-analyses of observational studies concluded that there were no associations between SSRI use during early (or anytime during) pregnancy and neonatal outcomes that were supported by convincing evidence. Only highly suggestive evidence supported an association between SSRI use in the first trimester and the risk for cardiovascular malformations; however, the studies included in the meta-analyses did not account for maternal diagnosis or severity of illness. The results of these studies suggest that any increase in the absolute risk of cardiac malformations with SSRI use during early pregnancy is small.

B – Incorrect. Meta-analysis and a recent large, population-based, cohort study indicate that there is no significant association between SSRI use in early pregnancy and risk of persistent pulmonary hypertension in offspring. However, there is a positive association between SSRI use in late pregnancy and risk of persistent pulmonary hypertension in offspring; clinically the absolute risk appears to be low.

C – Incorrect. After accounting for confounding factors (e.g., maternal severe psychiatric problems), first trimester exposure to antidepressants, including SSRIs (82%), compared with no exposure, was not associated with an increased risk for autism spectrum disorder, in a large retrospective cohort study. A recent meta-analysis of 14 studies that included maternal psychiatric disorders as covariates also concluded that there is no significant association between maternal SSRI use during any trimester of pregnancy and risk for autism spectrum disorder.

D – Incorrect.

E – Correct. Large cohort and case-controlled studies, as well as meta-analyses indicate there is no meaningful association between SSRI use during early pregnancy and risk for cardiovascular malformation, persistent pulmonary hypertension, or autism spectrum disorder in offspring.

References

Anderson KN, Lind JN, Simeone RM et al. Maternal use of specific antidepressant medications during early pregnancy and the risk of selected birth defects. *JAMA Psychiatry* 2020;77(12):1246–55.

Bérard A, Sheehy O, Zhao JP et al. SSRI and SNRI use during pregnancy and the risk of persistent pulmonary hypertension of the newborn. *Br J Clin Pharmacol* 2017;83(5):1126–33.

Biffi A, Cantarutti A, Rea F et al. Use of antidepressants during pregnancy and neonatal outcomes: an umbrella review of meta-analyses of observational studies. *J Psychiatr Res* 2020;124:99–108.

Grigoriadis S, Vonderporten EH, Mamisashvili L et al. Prenatal exposure to antidepressants and persistent pulmonary hypertension of the newborn: systematic review and meta-analysis. *BMJ* 2014;348:f6932.

Sujan AC, Rickert ME, Öberg AS et al. Associations of maternal antidepressant use during the first trimester of pregnancy with preterm birth, small for gestational age, autism spectrum disorder, and attention-deficit/hyperactivity disorder in offspring. *JAMA* 2017;317(15):1553–62.

Zhou XH, Li YJ, Ou JJ, Li YM. Association between maternal antidepressant use during pregnancy and autism spectrum disorder: an updated meta-analysis. *Mol Autism* 2018;9:21.

Unipolar Depression and Its Treatment

QUESTION TWENTY

Sasha is a 58-year-old patient with a history of depression who has been prescribed agomelatine. At present, she is relatively free of depressive symptoms, likely due in part to binding of agomelatine to what receptors in the suprachiasmatic nucleus?

A. Melatonin receptors

B. Serotonin 2C receptors

C. Melatonin and serotonin 2C receptors

Unipolar Depression and Its Treatment

Answer to Question Twenty

The correct answer is C.

Choice	Peer answers
Melatonin receptors	10%
Serotonin 2C receptors	19%
Melatonin and serotonin 2C receptors	70%

A and B – Partially correct.

C – Correct. Agomelatine is both a melatonin M1 and M2 receptor agonist and a serotonin 5HT2C receptor antagonist. This unique receptor profile gives agomelatine the ability to address impairments in neurotransmission as well as circadian rhythm dysfunction.

First, agomelatine can modulate circadian rhythms through its agonist actions at melatonin receptors. Melatonin is normally released from the pineal gland in response to environmental cues. It then acts on the suprachiasmatic nucleus, the location of the master clock, to reset circadian rhythms. Thus, as an agonist at melatonin receptors, agomelatine likewise regulates the molecular clock and can resynchronize circadian rhythms that are disturbed in depression.

Second, agomelatine affects neurotransmission by blocking 5HT2C receptors. Normally, serotonin excites GABA interneurons by stimulating 5HT2C receptors, which increases the release of the inhibitory neurotransmitter GABA. GABA can then bind to GABA-A receptors on noradrenergic and dopaminergic neurons. Since GABA is inhibitory, it will prevent these neurons from releasing norepinephrine and dopamine in the prefrontal cortex. As a 5HT2C receptor antagonist, agomelatine blocks serotonin from binding to GABA interneurons. This leads to disinhibition of monoaminergic neurons and increased norepinephrine and dopamine in the prefrontal cortex, which could potentially improve mood and cognition.

Reference
DeBodinat C, Guardiola-Lemaitre B, Mocaer E et al. Agomelatine, the first melatonergic antidepressant: discovery, characterization, and development. *Nat Rev Drug Discov* 2010;9:628–42.

QUESTION TWENTY-ONE

A patient presents to a new clinician with a major depressive episode. In addition to taking the patient's history, the two most useful factors for determining if a current depressive episode is indicative of unipolar or bipolar depression are:

A. Family history and input from someone close to the patient

B. Input from someone close to the patient and specific symptoms of the current episode

C. Specific symptoms of the current episode and patient insight

D. Patient insight and family history

Unipolar Depression and Its Treatment

Answer to Question Twenty-One

The correct answer is A.

Choice	Peer answers
Family history and input from someone close to the patient	68%
Input from someone close to the patient and specific symptoms of the current episode	15%
Specific symptoms of the current episode and patient insight	6%
Patient insight and family history	11%

A – Correct. Family history of bipolar disorders is arguably the most robust and reliable risk factor for bipolar disorder. Although most patients with bipolar disorder do not have a family history of bipolar disorder, individuals with a first-degree relative with bipolar disorder are at an 8–10 times greater risk of developing bipolar disorder compared to the general population. Obtaining additional information from a close outside informant, such as a parent or spouse, is also quite useful, as patients tend to under-report their hypomanic symptoms. Under-reporting may be due to patients not recalling important details of their history with enough accuracy or not viewing (hypo)manic symptoms as being problematic.

B – Partially correct.

C – Incorrect. Other than a history of a prior (hypo)manic episode, patients with unipolar depressive episodes are diagnosed using the same symptom criteria as patients with bipolar depressive episodes; thus, specific symptoms during the current episode may not help differentiate between unipolar depression and bipolar disorder. An exception would be a major depressive episode with mixed features, which may indicate a bipolar disorder. Patient insight may not be a reliable factor for differentiating between unipolar or bipolar depression because patients may not recall important details of their history with enough accuracy or may not view previous (hypo)manic symptoms as being problematic.

D – Partially correct.

References

Angst J, **Azorin JM**, **Bowden CL** et al. Prevalence and characteristics of undiagnosed bipolar disorders in patients with a major depressive episode: the BRIDGE study. *Arch Gen Psychiatry* 2011;68(8):791–8.

Perlis RH, Brown E, Baker RW, Nierenberg AA. Clinical features of bipolar depression versus major depressive disorder in large multicenter trials. *Am J Psychiatry* 2006;163(2):225–31.

Stahl SM. *Stahl's essential psychopharmacology*, fifth edition. New York, NY: Cambridge University Press; 2021. (Chapter 6)

Unipolar Depression and Its Treatment

QUESTION TWENTY-TWO

April is a 14-year-old patient recently diagnosed with moderate to severe major depressive disorder (MDD). She endorses passive suicidal ideation, but no specific plan or intention for suicide attempt. She denies any suicidal ideation or attempts prior to her current depressive episode. In addition to beginning cognitive behavioral therapy (CBT), which pharmacotherapy option would be best suited for treating her depressive episode?

A. Imipramine

B. Bupropion

C. Fluoxetine

D. No pharmacotherapy should be initiated

Unipolar Depression and Its Treatment

Answer to Question Twenty-Two

The correct answer is C.

Choice	Peer answers
Imipramine	1%
Bupropion	6%
Fluoxetine	87%
No pharmacotherapy should be initiated	6%

A – Incorrect. Randomized clinical trials suggest tricyclic antidepressants (TCAs), including imipramine, are not useful for treating depression in children and only marginally effective in adolescents. TCAs are not recommended as first-line pharmacotherapy for the treatment of pediatric MDD.

B – Incorrect. To date, there are no randomized clinical trials examining safety or efficacy of bupropion in pediatric MDD.

C – Correct. Fluoxetine, a selective serotonin reuptake inhibitor (SSRI), has a good evidence base for efficacy in treating pediatric MDD and is one of only two antidepressants with US Food and Drug Administration (FDA) approval for pediatric MDD. Escitalopram, also an SSRI, is the second antidepressant approved for treating pediatric MDD. There is no strong evidence to suggest that any particular SSRI is more effective than any other for pediatric MDD. However, both the National Institute for Health and Care Excellence (NICE) and the American Academy of Child and Adolescent Psychiatry (AACAP) recommend evidence-based psychotherapy, such as CBT, and/or fluoxetine to treat moderate to severe depression in adolescence.

D – Incorrect. Although there are several antidepressant clinical trials reporting negative findings in pediatric MDD, specifically industry-sponsored trials, these trials suffer from implementation challenges (i.e., study design) and should be considered failed trials. By contrast, trials funded by the National Institute of Mental Health, which are characterized by methodological strengths and lower placebo response rates, demonstrate good efficacy of SSRIs for treating pediatric depression. Concerns regarding an increased risk for suicide with SSRI use in pediatric MDD may not warrant avoidance of pharmacotherapy. Adding fluoxetine to CBT appears to eliminate fluoxetine-associated risk for suicidal events. Furthermore, epidemiological data suggest that youth with depression receiving antidepressants are at lower risk for death by suicide than untreated youth.

References

Birmaher B, Brent D, AACAP Work Group on Quality Issues et al. Practice parameter for the assessment and treatment of children and adolescents with depressive disorders. *J Am Acad Child Adolesc Psychiatry* 2007;46(11):1503–26.

Dwyer JB, Stringaris A, Brent DA, Bloch MH. Annual research review: defining and treating pediatric treatment-resistant depression. *J Child Psychol Psychiatry* 2020;61(3):312–32.

Giles LL, Martini DR. Challenges and promises of pediatric psychopharmacology. *Acad Pediatr* 2016;16(6):508–18.

National Institute for Health and Care Excellence. Depression in children and young people: identification and management. NICE guideline [NG134]. 2019. Available at: www.nice.org.uk/guidance/ng134.

Walkup JT. Antidepressant efficacy for depression in children and adolescents: industry- and NIMH-funded studies. *Am J Psychiatry* 2017;174(5):430–7.

Unipolar Depression and Its Treatment

QUESTION TWENTY-THREE

The hypothesis that the therapeutic effects of antidepressants are due to downstream changes in neuroplasticity is consistent with the fact that clinical improvement with antidepressants is typically delayed by several weeks. The downstream effects of monoamine antidepressants include:

A. Decreased AMPA receptor expression, decreased NMDA receptor expression, decreased glutamate

B. Increased AMPA receptor expression, decreased NMDA receptor expression, decreased glutamate

C. Decreased AMPA receptor expression, increased NMDA receptor expression, decreased glutamate

D. Increased AMPA receptor expression, decreased NMDA receptor expression, increased glutamate

Unipolar Depression and Its Treatment

Answer to Question Twenty-Three

The correct answer is B.

Choice	Peer answers
Decreased AMPA receptor expression, decreased NMDA receptor expression, decreased glutamate	8%
Increased AMPA receptor expression, decreased NMDA receptor expression, decreased glutamate	43%
Decreased AMPA receptor expression, increased NMDA receptor expression, decreased glutamate	21%
Increased AMPA receptor expression, decreased NMDA receptor expression, increased glutamate	29%

A – Incorrect. AMPA receptor expression is increased.

B – Correct. There is increasing evidence that the underlying mechanism of antidepressant treatment may not be alterations in the levels of monoamines themselves, but rather changes in the downstream molecular events and neuroplasticity triggered by those monoamines. Monoaminergic antidepressants likely exert their therapeutic effects by influencing downstream signaling, such as increased α-amino-3-hydroxy-5-methyl-4-isoxazolepropionic acid, or AMPA, receptor expression, decreased N-methyl-D-aspartate, or NMDA, receptor expression, and decreased glutamate, suggesting agents with direct activity at these downstream targets may lead to faster treatment response. Antidepressant treatments may modify the AMPA:NMDA receptor ratio, resulting in downregulated NMDA receptors, and increased AMPA receptors.

C – Incorrect. NMDA receptor expression is decreased.

D – Incorrect. Glutamate is decreased.

References

Abdallah CG, Adams TG, Kelmendi B, et al. Ketamine's mechanism of action: a path to rapid-acting antidepressants. *Depress Anxiety* 2016;33(8):689–97.

Barbon A, Caracciolo L, Orlandi C, et al. Chronic antidepressant treatments induce a time-dependent up-regulation of AMPA receptor subunit protein levels. *Neurochem Int* 2011;59(6):896–905.

Bunney BG, Bunney WE. Rapid-acting antidepressant strategies: mechanisms of action. *Int J Neuropsychopharmacol* 2012;15(5):695–713.

Racagni G, Popoli M. Cellular and molecular mechanisms in the long-term action of antidepressants. *Dialogues Clin Neurosci* 2008;10(4):385–400.

Stahl SM. *Stahl's Essential Psychopharmacology*, fourth edition. New York, NY: Cambridge University Press; 2013. (Chapter 6)

CHAPTER PEER COMPARISON

For the Unipolar Depression section, the correct answer was selected 71% of the time.

BOOK PEER COMPARISON

For *Stahl's Self-Assessment Examination in Psychiatry; Multiple Choice Questions for Clinicians, Fourth Edition*, the correct answer was selected 68% of the time.

Unipolar Depression and Its Treatment

INDEX

Index

Index

Index